Periease

D
UnivIA

UMass Memorial Medical Center
Professor of Medicine
University of Massachusetts Medical School, Worcester, MA

JONES AND BARTLETT PUBLISHERS

World Headquarters

Jones and Bartlett Publishers	Jones and Bartlett Publishers	Jones and Bartlett Publishers
40 Tall Pine Drive	Canada	International
Sudbury, MA 01776	6339 Ormindale Way	Barb House, Barb Mews
978-443-5000	Mississauga, Ontario L5V 1J2	London W6 7PA
info@jbpub.com	Canada	United Kingdom
www.jbpub.com		

Jones and Bartlett's books and products are available through most bookstores and online booksellers. To contact Jones and Bartlett Publishers directly, call 800-832-0034, fax 978-443-8000, or visit our website, www.jbpub.com.

Substantial discounts on bulk quantities of Jones and Bartlett's publications are available to corporations, professional associations, and other qualified organizations. For details and specific discount information, contact the special sales department at Jones and Bartlett via the above contact information or send an email to specialsales@jbpub.com.

The authors, editor, and publisher have made every effort to provide accurate information. However, they are not responsible for errors, omissions, or for any outcomes related to the use of the contents of this book and take no responsibility for the use of the products and procedures described. Treatments and side effects described in this book may not be applicable to all people; likewise, some people may require a dose or experience a side effect that is not described herein. Drugs and medical devices are discussed that may have limited availability controlled by the Food and Drug Administration (FDA) for use only in a research study or clinical trial. Research, clinical practice, and government regulations often change the accepted standard in this field. When consideration is being given to use of any drug in the clinical setting, the healthcare provider or reader is responsible for determining FDA status of the drug, reading the package insert, and reviewing prescribing information for the most up-to-date recommendations on dose, precautions, and contraindications, and determining the appropriate usage for the product. This is especially important in the case of drugs that are new or seldom used.

Production Credits
Senior Acquisitions Editor: Alison Hankey
Senior Editorial Assistant: Jessica Acox
Production Director: Amy Rose
Associate Production Editor: Laura Almozara
Senior Marketing Manager: Barb Bartoszek
V.P., Manufacturing and Inventory Control:
   Therese Connell
Composition: diacriTech, Chennai, India
Printing and Binding: Malloy, Inc.
Cover Printing: Malloy, Inc.

Cover Credits
Cover Images: Abstract vessel: © Alexfiodorov/
   Dreamstime.com, Abstract blood cells: © Benjamin
   Haas/Dreamstime.com, Abstract inside of vein:
   © Sebastian Kaulitzki/Dreamstime.com, Blood cells:
   © Andreus/Dreamstime.com, Vein system: © Aleksandr
   Frolov/Dreamstime.com, Running man: © Sebastian
   Kaultizki/Dreamstime.com
Cover Design: Kristin E. Parker

Library of Congress Cataloging-in-Publication Data
Alonso, Alvaro, 1977
   Peripheral vascular disease/Alvaro Alonso, David McManus, Daniel Z. Fisher.
      p. ; cm.
   Includes bibliographical references and index.
   ISBN-13: 978-0-7637-5538-6
   ISBN-10: 0-7637-5538-9
   1. Peripheral vascular diseases–Handbooks, manuals, etc. 2. Arteries–Diseases–Handbooks, manuals, etc. I. McManus, David. II. Fisher, Daniel Z. III. Title.
   [DNLM: 1. Peripheral Vascular Diseases–diagnosis–Handbooks. 2. Peripheral Vascular Diseases–therapy–Handbooks. WG 39 A454d 2011]
   RC694.A46 2011
   616.1'3–dc22
                           2009045709
6048

Printed in the United States of America
14 13 12 11 10   10 9 8 7 6 5 4 3 2 1

DEDICATION

To Alejandra. To my parents and professors. To our patients,
who deserve our best efforts and compassion.
Alvaro Alonso, MD

To my wife.
David D. McManus, MD

To Carol, Michael, Alison, and Emily.
Daniel Z. Fisher, MD, MPh

Contents

Editor's Preface

Diseases of the peripheral arteries affect a great number of adults. While atherosclerosis is clinically the most common process encountered, other disorders such as inflammation, aneurysms, and dysplasia may involve the peripheral arteries. Due to its protean manifestations, peripheral vascular disease is likely to be encountered by physicians practicing in many disciplines. In this book, Drs. Alonso, McManus, and Fisher describe the common diseases affecting the arteries that supply the various vascular beds. The authors use a concise and focused format to present the clinical manifestations, diagnostic evaluation, and evidence-based therapeutic considerations. The text is supplemented by many informative tables and illustrations. Well-reproduced images illustrate important clinical points and a pertinent list of references is included. The authors are to be congratulated for sharing their vast expertise in this field and for producing a concise, yet very informative and balanced manuscript. Any healthcare professional who cares for patients with risk factors for cardiac disease or vascular insufficiency will find this book to be most useful in their practice.

Dennis A. Tighe, MD, FACP, FACC
Worcester, MA

Preface

Peripheral arterial disease (PAD) affects a large portion of our patient population. It is a major cause of morbidity and mortality, and its burden is increasing worldwide. Despite this, PAD remains a disease with which many clinicians are unfamiliar. When we were invited to author this book, we thought that it would be a wonderful and challenging opportunity to summarize the literature in such a manner that medical audiences of different backgrounds and training levels could understand it and apply resources adequately to benefit individual patients.

Our goal was simple: To provide a synopsis of PAD that was concise, unbiased, and comprehensive. One of the major challenges was dealing with paucity of data, and the ever-changing and controversial nature of many of the diagnostic and treatment modalities. We provide a description of relevant vascular anatomy and pathophysiology. We also provide a focused review of diagnostic modalities used in screening for PAD and contemporary medical and interventional treatments used for PAD. We have summarized the data using bullet points, condensed tables, high-quality figures, and diagrams, with the goal of making our work easy to access for busy clinicians and students.

We are certain readers will find this book a useful tool that will deepen their knowledge of this fascinating area of medicine.

Acknowledgments

We are very thankful for the extraordinary images obtained with the help of the following persons:

- Denise Kush, RDMS, RVT, and the staff of the Vascular Laboratory, UMass Memorial Health Care
- Andres Schanzer, MD, Assistant Professor of Surgery, University of Massachusetts Medical Center and Medical School
- David J. Sheehan, DO, Department of Radiology, University of Massachusetts Medical Center and Medical School
- Raul Galvez, MD, MPH, and Hale Ersoy, MD, Department of Radiology, Brigham and Women's Hospital, Harvard Medical School

CHAPTER 1

Vascular Biology of Atherosclerosis

INTRODUCTION

Atherosclerosis is defined as a form of arteriosclerosis (abnormal thickening and hardening of the arterial walls with loss of elasticity) characterized by atheromatous deposits and fibrosis of the inner layer of the arteries (the intima). Its clinical manifestations are well known and include coronary heart disease, stroke, and peripheral vascular disease.[1, 2]

PATHOGENESIS

Atherosclerotic lesions progress from a variety of pathogenic factors that impact the vascular wall.

Endothelial Dysfunction

Endothelial dysfunction and impaired vascular reactivity can be induced by dyslipidemia and is more prominent in patients with a family history of coronary heart disease or diabetes.[3, 4]

Endothelial dysfunction is induced by oxidized LDL,[5] worsened by cigarette smoking, and can be reversed with treatment of hyperlipidemia by diet or statin therapy (acting by increasing the bioavailability of nitric oxide),[6, 7] ACE inhibitors,[8] or with antioxidants such as vitamin C or flavonoids contained in red wine and purple grape juice (Table 1.1).[9, 10]

Dyslipidemia

It is well known that lipid abnormalities are extremely important in the development of atherosclerosis, in particular, high levels of low-density lipoprotein (LDL) and low levels of high-density lipoprotein (HDL).[11, 12]

Circulating LDL rapidly accumulates in the cholesterol-enriched macrophages (called foam cells), but not in the lipid core.[13] LDL needs to be oxidized to allow uptake by macrophages via "scavenger receptors" (e.g., CD36).[14] Macrophage uptake of LDL cholesterol may initially be an adaptive response, preventing oxidized-LDL-induced endothelial injury. However, cholesterol accumulation in foam cells leads to mitochondrial dysfunction, apoptosis, and necrosis, with resultant release of cellular proteases, inflammatory cytokines, and prothrombotic molecules (Figure 1.1).[15]

Table 1.1   Factors that Cause and Interventions that Improve Endothelial Dysfunction

FACTORS ASSOCIATED WITH ENDOTHELIAL DYSFUNCTION	INTERVENTIONS THAT IMPROVE ENDOTHELIAL FUNCTION
Increased age	L-arginine
Male sex	Estrogen
Family history of coronary heart disease	Antioxidants
Smoking	Smoking cessation
Increased-serum LDL cholesterol	Cholesterol lowering
Low-serum HDL cholesterol	Statins
Hypertension	ACE inhibitors
Increased-serum homocysteine	Exercise
Diabetes mellitus	Homocysteine lowering
Obesity	Flavonoids
High-fat meal	

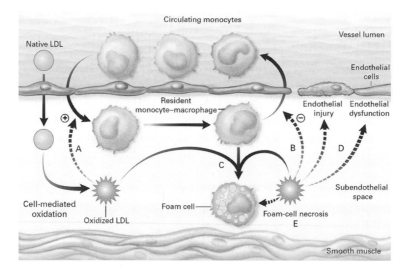

Figure 1.1

Early Events in Atherogenesis. Native LDL becomes trapped in the subendothelial space, where it can be oxidized by resident vascular cells such as smooth-muscle cells, endothelial cells, and macrophages. Oxidized LDL stimulates (plus sign) monocyte chemotaxis (A) and inhibits (minus sign) monocyte egress from the vascular wall (B). Monocytes differentiate into macrophages that internalize oxidized LDL, leading to foam-cell formation (C). Oxidized LDL also causes endothelial dysfunction and injury (D), as well as foam-cell necrosis (E), resulting in the release of lysosomal enzymes and necrotic debris. Broken arrows indicate adverse effects of oxidized LDL. Reproduced as depicted (modified) in N Engl J Med 1997;337:408 with permission from the authors of the original figure (holders of the Copyright): Steinberg D, et al. Oxidatively modified low density lipoproteins: a potential role in recruitment and retention of monocyte/macrophages during atherogenesis. Proc Natl Acad Sci U S A. 1987;84:2995–2998.

Oxidized LDL also disrupts endothelial cell surface and may play a role in plaque instability. Levels of oxidized LDL are increased in patients with an acute coronary syndrome and correlate with its severity.[16, 17]

In contrast, HDL has anti-atherogenic properties, including reverse cholesterol transport, maintenance of endothelial function, protection against thrombosis, and decreased blood viscosity. There is an inverse relationship between HDL cholesterol levels and cardiovascular risk.[11]

The role of hypertriglyceridemia is less clear, because confirmation of its specific role is made difficult by its association with low-serum HDL.[18]

Lipoprotein(a) also binds to macrophages and leads to foam cell formation.[19]

Inflammation

The presence of inflammation due to both cellular and humoral pathways has been well described.[20] Macrophages loaded with oxidized LDL release cytokines that further perpetuate the cycle of inflammation and endothelial cell injury.[21] These cytokines include interleukins, tumor necrosis factor alpha, intercellular adhesion molecule 1, monocyte chemotactic protein 1, granulocyte-macrophage colony stimulating factors, and soluble CD40 ligand. These cytokines induce reactive oxygen species and induce cell injury (Figure 1.1).[20]

Markers of increased systemic inflammation are directly associated with the risk of atherosclerosis. Serum C–reactive protein is a marker of atherosclerotic cardiovascular risk.[20]

Tissue Factor

Tissue factor is the primary initiator of coagulation and is found in the atherosclerotic plaque. It not only contributes to the development of thrombosis following plaque rupture, but also accelerates endothelial regrowth over the plaque after rupture.[22]

Angiotensin II

Angiotensin II promotes the development and severity of atherosclerosis. It also plays a role in the modulation of vascular smooth muscle cell proliferation and the production of extracellular matrix.[23]

Endothelin-1

Oxidized LDL also stimulates the production of Endothelin-1, a potent vasoconstrictor and a mitogen for vascular smooth muscle cells.[24]

Flow Characteristics

Hemodynamic shear stress plays a particularly important role in the development of atherosclerotic peripheral arterial disease (PAD). Plaques typically occur at branch points, where blood must undergo a change in velocity and direction. Decreased shear stress resulting from disrupted laminar blood flow appears to result in atherogenesis at these sites as a result of increased turbulence, repetitive vascular injury, altered endothelial cell function, enhanced monocyte binding, and LDL accumulation.[21, 25]

Plaque Hemorrhage

As the atherosclerotic plaque expands, it acquires its own expanded vasa vasorum. These vessels, however, are prone to disruption, leading to hemorrhage within the plaque.[26] Plaque hemorrhage may contribute to the progression of atherosclerosis.[27]

Plaque Rupture

Atherosclerosis is generally asymptomatic until the plaque stenosis produces a critical reduction in blood flow. However, acute coronary and cerebrovascular syndromes (unstable angina, myocardial infarction, sudden death, and stroke) are typically due to rupture of plaques with less than 50% stenosis.[28, 29] Plaque rupture may also be silent. Repeated cycles of silent plaque rupture, thrombosis, and wound healing may cause progression of atherosclerosis by increasing the plaque burden.[30]

Infection

Chronic infection has been suggested as a possible contributing factor of atherosclerosis. It could act by a number of mechanisms, including direct vascular injury and induction of a systemic inflammatory state. Although controversial, organisms implicated include *Chlamydia pneumoniae*, cytomegalovirus, *Helicobacter pylori*, enterovirus, hepatitis A virus, herpes simplex virus, and human immunodeficiency virus.[20, 31, 32]

Figure 1.2 is a representative diagram of the steps in the development of atherosclerosis.

HISTOLOGY

The initial lesion in atherosclerosis involves the intima of the artery and begins in childhood with the development of fatty streaks (Table 1.2).[33] The advanced lesions of atherosclerosis occur more frequently in older individuals.[34–36] Early arterial accumulation of cholesterol causes a reduction in arterial distensibility, which occurs before other vessel-wall changes become apparent.[37]

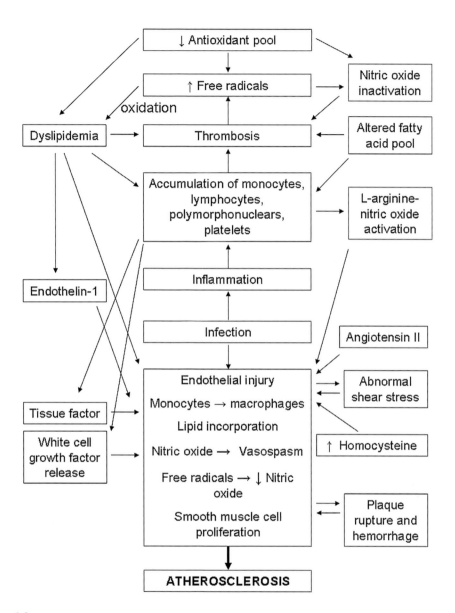

Figure 1.2

Postulated steps in the pathogenesis of atherosclerosis.

Reprinted from: J Am Coll Cardiol, Vol. 31, Rand JL, Saldeen TG, Mehta K. Interactive role of infection, inflammation and traditional risk factors in atherosclerosis and coronary artery disease, Page 1217, Copyright, 1998, with permission from Elsevier.

Table 1.2   American Heart Association Lesion Classification System and Correspondence with Classification of Gross Arterial Specimens

AHA Grade	Criteria	Comments and Corresponding Gross Classification
0	Normal artery with or without adaptive intimal thickening	Normal tissue
1	Isolated MFCs containing lipid; no extracellular lipid; variable adaptive intimal thickening grossly with lipid staining	Initial atherosclerotic lesion, sometimes visible grossly with lipid staining
2	Numerous MFCs, often in layers, with fine particles of extracellular lipid; no distinct pools of extracellular lipid: variable adaptive intimal thickening	Fatty streak, visible grossly with lipid staining
3	Numerous MFCs with $\geq$ pools of extracellular lipid; no well-defined core of extracellular lipid	Fatty plaque, raised fatty streak, intermediate lesion, or transitional lesion
4	Numerous MFGs plus well-defined core of extracellular lipid, but with luminal surface covered by relatively normal intima	Atheroma, fibrous plaque, or raised lesion
5	Numerous MFCs, well-defined core or multiple cores of extracellular lipid, plus reactive fibrotic cap, vascularization, or calcium	Fibroatheroma, fibrous plaque, or raised lesion
6	All of the above plus surface defect, hematoma, hemorrhage, or thrombosis	Complicated lesion

Key: MFC, macrophage foam cell. Table adapted from reference 34.

Fatty Streaks

The first phase in atherosclerosis histologically presents as focal thickening of the intima, with an increase in smooth muscle cells and extracellular matrix.[38] These smooth muscle cells (possibly derived from hematopoietic stem cells) migrate and proliferate within the intima.[39] This is followed by accumulation of intra- and extracellular lipid deposits, macrophages, and T lymphocytes.[20]

As these lesions increase in size, smooth muscle cells are susceptible to apoptosis, which triggers further macrophage infiltration and cytoplasmic remnants that can calcify, perhaps contributing to the transition of fatty streaks into atherosclerotic plaques.[40]

Fibrous Plaque

The fatty streak evolves into the fibrous plaque via accumulation of connective tissue with an increased number of smooth muscle cells with increased intra- and extracellular lipid content.[34]

Advanced Lesions

More advanced lesions tend to become revascularized from both the luminal and medial aspects, but often the core is necrotic and rich in lipid contents, which over time can become calcified.[34] Advanced lesions are associated with arterial remodeling (Figure 1.3).[41] Positive remodeling is present when a compensatory increase in local vessel size appears in response to increasing plaque burden, while negative remodeling is present when there is a smaller vessel size due to a smaller external elastic membrane area at the lesion site. Positive remodeling is commonly encountered with complex, unstable plaques. Negative remodeling, on the other hand, is associated with smoother, stable plaques.[42]

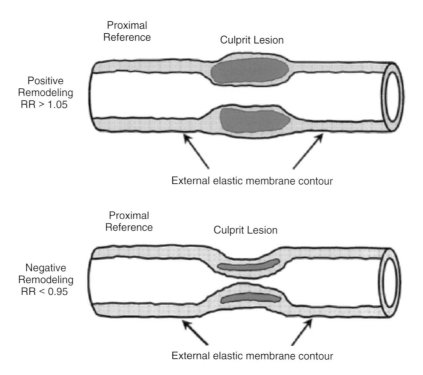

Figure 1.3

Positive and negative arterial remodeling. Diagrams of longitudinal sections through vessel segments with positively and negatively remodeled lesions are shown. Remodeling ratio (RR) = external elastic membrane area lesion/external elastic membrane area proximal reference.

Reprinted from: J Am Coll Cardiol, Vol. 38, Zchoenhagen P, Ziada KM, Vince DG, Nissen SE, Tuzcu EM. Arterial remodeling and coronary artery disease: the concept of "dilated" versus "obstructive" coronary atherosclerosis, Page 297, Copyright, 2001, with permission from Elsevier.

◇◇◇◇◇◇◇◇◇◇◇◇

REFERENCES

1. Hansson GK. Inflammation, atherosclerosis and coronary artery disease. *N Engl J Med.* 2005;352:1685–1695.
2. Faxon DP, Fuster V, Libby P, et al. Atherosclerotic vascular disease conference: writing group III: pathophysiology. *Circulation.* 2004;109:2617–2625.
3. Schachinger V, Britten MB, Elsner M, Walter DH, Scharrer I, Zeiher AM. A positive family history of premature coronary artery disease is associated with impaired endothelium-dependent coronary blood flow regulation. *Circulation.* 1999;100:1502–1508.
4. Balletshofer BM, Rittig K, Enderle MD, et al. Endothelial dysfunction is detectable in young normotensive first-degree relatives of subjects with type 2 diabetes in association with insulin resistance. *Circulation.* 2000;101:1780–1784.
5. Anderson TJ, Meredith IT, Charbonneau F, et al. Endothelium-dependent coronary vasomotion relates to the susceptibility of LDL to oxidation in humans. *Circulation.* 1996;93:1647–1650.
6. Harrison DG, Armstrong ML, Freiman PC, Heistad DD. Restoration of endothelium-dependent relaxation by dietary treatment of atherosclerosis. *J Clin Invest.* 1987;80:1808–1811.
7. John S, Schlaich M, Langenfeld M, et al. Increased bioavailability of nitric oxide after lipid-lowering therapy in hypercholesterolemic patients: a randomized, placebo-controlled, double-blind study. *Circulation.* 1998;98:211–216.
8. Mancini GB, Henry GC, Macaya C, et al. Angiotensin-converting enzyme inhibition with quinapril improves endothelial vasomotor dysfunction in patients with coronary artery disease: the TREND (Trial on Reversing ENdothelial Dysfunction) study. *Circulation.* 1996;94:258–265.
9. Levine GN, Frei B, Koulouris SN, Gerhard MD, Keaney JF, Jr, Vita JA. Ascorbic acid reverses endothelial vasomotor dysfunction in patients with coronary artery disease. *Circulation.* 1996;93:1107–1113.
10. Stein JH, Keevil JG, Wiebe DA, Aeschlimann S, Folts JD. Purple grape juice improves endothelial function and reduces the susceptibility of LDL cholesterol to oxidation in patients with coronary artery disease. *Circulation.* 1999;100:1050–1055.
11. Coonet MT, Dudina A, De Bacquer D, et al. HDL cholesterol protects against cardiovascular disease in both genders, at all ages and at all levels of risk. *Atherosclerosis.* 2009;206:611–616.
12. Expert Panel on Detection, Evaluation, and Treatment of High Blood Cholesterol in Adults. Executive Summary of the Third Report of the National Cholesterol Education Program (NCEP) Expert Panel on Detection, Evaluation, and Treatment of High Blood Cholesterol in Adults (Adult Treatment Panel III). *JAMA.* 2001;285:2486–2497.
13. Iuliano L, Mauriello A, Sbarigia E, Spagnoli LG, Violi F. Radiolabeled native low-density lipoprotein injected into patients with carotid stenosis accumulates in macrophages of atherosclerotic plaque: effect of vitamin E supplementation. *Circulation.* 2000;101:1249–1254.
14. Podrez EA, Febbraio M, Sheibani N, et al. Macrophage scavenger receptor CD36 is the major receptor for LDL modified by monocyte-generated reactive nitrogen species. *J Clin Invest.* 2000;105:1095–1108.
15. Tabas I. Consequences of cellular cholesterol accumulation: basic concepts and physiological implications. *J Clin Invest.* 2002;110:905–911.
16. Ehara S, Ueda M, Naruko T, et al. Elevated levels of oxidized low density lipoprotein show a positive relationship with the severity of acute coronary syndromes. *Circulation.* 2001;103:1955–1960.
17. Tsimikas S, Bergmark C, Beyer RW, et al. Temporal increases in plasma markers of oxidized low-density lipoprotein strongly reflect the presence of acute coronary syndromes. *J Am Coll Cardiol.* 2003;41:360–370.
18. Walter M, Le N. The role of hypertriglyceridemia in atherosclerosis. *Curr Atheroscler Rep.* 2007;9:110.
19. Marcovina SM, Koschinsky ML. Lipoprotein(a) as a risk factor for coronary artery disease. *Am J Cardiol.* 1998;82:57.
20. Libby P, Ridker PM, Maseri A. Inflammation and atherosclerosis. *Circulation.* 2002;105:1135–1143.
21. Berliner JA, Navab M, Fogelman AM, et al. Atherosclerosis: basic mechanisms. Oxidation, inflammation, and genetics. *Circulation.* 1995;91:2488–2496.
22. Hasenstab D, Lea H, Hart CE, Lok S, Clowes AW. Tissue factor overexpression in rat arterial neointima models thrombosis and progression of advanced atherosclerosis. *Circulation.* 2000;101:2651–2657.
23. Potter DD, Sobey CG, Tompkins PK, Rossen JD, Heistad DD. Evidence that macrophages in atherosclerotic lesions contain angiotensin II. *Circulation.* 1998;98:800–807.

24. Mathew V, Cannan CR, Miller VM, et al. Enhanced endothelin-mediated coronary vasoconstriction and attenuated basal nitric oxide activity in experimental hypercholesterolemia. *Circulation*. 1997;96: 1930–1936.

25. Hagiwara H, Mitsumata M, Yamane T, Jin X, Yoshida Y. Laminar shear stress-induced GRO mRNA and protein expression in endothelial cells. *Circulation*. 1998;98:2584–2590.

26. Virmani R, Narula J, Farb A. When neoangiogenesis ricochets. *Am Heart J*. 1998;136:937–939.

27. Kolodgie FD, Gold HK, Burke AP, et al. Intraplaque hemorrhage and progression of coronary atheroma. *N Engl J Med*. 2003;349:2316–2325.

28. Falk E, Shah PK, Fuster V. Coronary plaque disruption. *Circulation*. 1995;92:657–671.

29. Little WC, Constantinescu M, Applegate RJ, et al. Can coronary angiography predict the site of a subsequent myocardial infarction in patients with mild-to-moderate coronary artery disease? *Circulation*. 1988;78:1157–1166.

30. Burke AP, Kolodgie FD, Farb A, et al. Healed plaque ruptures and sudden coronary death: evidence that subclinical rupture has a role in plaque progression. *Circulation*. 2001;103:934–940.

31. Mahmoudi M, Curzen N, Gallagher PJ. Atherogenesis: the role of inflammation and infection. *Histopathology*. 2007;50:535.

32. Barbaro G. Vascular injury, hypertension and coronary artery disease in human immunodeficiency virus infection. *Clin Ter*. 2008;159:51.

33. Strong JP, Malcom GT, McMahan CA, et al. Prevalence and extent of atherosclerosis in adolescents and young adults: implications for prevention from the Pathobiological Determinants of Atherosclerosis in Youth Study. *JAMA*. 1999;281:727–735.

34. Stary HC, Chandler AB, Dinsmore RE, et al. A definition of advanced types of atherosclerotic lesions and a histological classification of atherosclerosis: a report from the Committee on Vascular Lesions of the Council on Arteriosclerosis, American Heart Association. *Circulation*. 1995;92:1355–1374.

35. Tuzcu EM, Kapadia SR, Tutar E, et al. High prevalence of coronary atherosclerosis in asymptomatic teenagers and young adults: evidence from intravascular ultrasound. *Circulation*. 2001;103:2705–2710.

36. McGill HC, Jr, McMahan CA, Zieske AW, et al. Association of Coronary Heart Disease risk factors with microscopic qualities of coronary atherosclerosis in youth. *Circulation*. 2000;102:374–379.

37. Dart AM, Lacombe F, Yeoh JK, et al. Aortic distensibility in patients with isolated hypercholesterolaemia, coronary artery disease, or cardiac transplant. *Lancet*. 1991;338:270–273.

38. Davies MJ, Woolf N, Rowles PM, Pepper J. Morphology of the endothelium over atherosclerotic plaques in human coronary arteries. *Br Heart J*. 1988;60: 459–464.

39. Sata M, Saiura A, Kunisato A, et al. Hematopoietic stem cells differentiate into vascular cells that participate in the pathogenesis of atherosclerosis. *Nat Med*. 2002;8:403–409.

40. Kockx MM, De Meyer GR, Muhring J, Jacob W, Bult H, Herman AG. Apoptosis and related proteins in different stages of human atherosclerotic plaques. *Circulation*. 1998;97:2307–2315.

41. Schoenhagen P, Ziada KM, Vince DG, Nissen SE, Tuzcu EM. Arterial remodeling and coronary artery disease: the concept of "dilated" versus "obstructive" coronary atherosclerosis. *J Am Coll Cardiol*. 2001;38:297–306.

42. Schoenhagen P, Ziada KM, Kapadia SR, Crowe TD, Nissen SE, Tuzcu EM. Extent and direction of arterial remodeling in stable versus unstable coronary syndromes: an intravascular ultrasound study. *Circulation*. 2000;101:598–603.

CHAPTER 2

Peripheral Arterial Disease of the Lower Extremities

ANATOMY

The abdominal aorta most commonly divides at the level of the fourth lumbar vertebra into the two common iliac arteries. The common iliac artery then divides into the external iliac and internal iliac (hypogastric) arteries. The external iliac artery supplies the lower extremity, whereas the hypogastric artery supplies the buttock, viscera of the pelvis, the medial thigh, as well as either the uterus and vagina or the testicles and penis (Figure 2.1).

The external iliac artery passes downward from the medial aspect of the psoas muscle to the inguinal ligament, midway between the anterior superior iliac crest and the symphysis pubis, where it enters the thigh and becomes the common femoral artery.

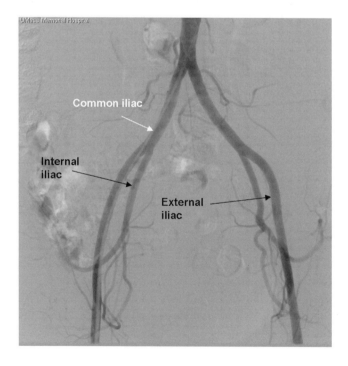

Figure 2.1

Angiogram of the iliac arteries.

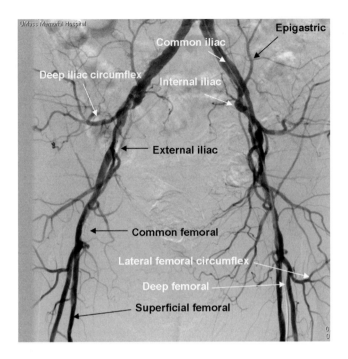

Figure 2.2

Angiogram of the main iliofemoral vessels.

The external iliac gives off two branches, the inferior (or deep) epigastric artery and the deep iliac circumflex (Figure 2.2).

The common femoral artery courses caudally until it divides into the superficial and deep (profunda) femoral arteries. The deep femoral artery usually arises 4 cm below the inguinal ligament and courses laterally. The superficial femoral artery courses caudally and medially until it crosses the medial aspect of the femur in the middle third of the thigh (Figure 2.3). At this point the superficial femoral artery enters the adductor canal (Hunter's canal). The only major branch of the superficial femoral is the superior geniculate artery. The deep femoral artery gives off the lateral circumflex femoral, the medial circumflex femoral, and the perforating arteries. These branches often anastomose with branches of the internal iliac artery to provide collateral circulation in the presence of external iliac occlusion.

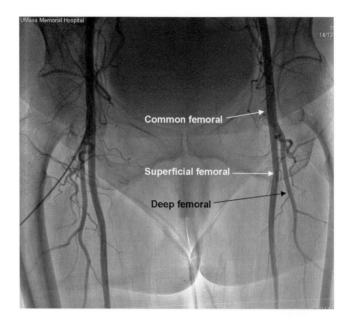

Figure 2.3

Angiogram of the femoral artery bifurcation.

The superficial femoral artery becomes the popliteal artery after it exits the inferior aspect of the adductor canal. The popliteal artery extends downward to the most caudal portion of the popliteus muscle, where it divides into the anterior tibial artery and the tibio-peroneal trunk. At the knee, the popliteal artery gives rise to the genicular arteries and the sural arteries.

The anterior tibial artery supplies the anterior aspect of the lower leg and extends into the dorsum of the foot as the dorsalis pedis artery. The anterior tibial recurrent artery courses cranially to connect with the genicular network. The posterior tibial artery arises off the tibio-peroneal trunk and supplies the posterior portion of the lower leg. The posterior tibial artery gives rise to the fibular artery, which forms an anastamosis with the genicular network. The third main branch of the lower leg, arising off the tibio-peroneal trunk, is the peroneal artery. The peroneal artery gives rise to perforating branches above the ankle that communicate with the distal portions of the anterior and posterior tibial arteries (Figure 2.4).

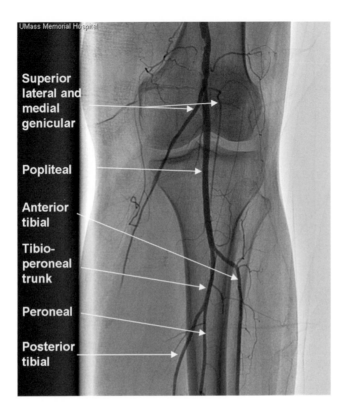

Figure 2.4

Angiogram of the femoral-popliteal bifurcation and its branches.

The posterior tibial artery branches at the level of the hindfoot to the medial and lateral plantar arteries. The dorsalis pedis artery branches to the lateral and medial tarsal arteries, the arcade artery, and the plantar arch (Figure 2.5).

PATHOPHYSIOLOGY

The term peripheral arterial disease (PAD) is conventionally used to describe atherosclerotic lesions that result in obstructed blood flow to the lower or upper extremities. While non-atherosclerotic causes of PAD should be understood and considered (Table 2.1), they represent the vast minority of cases. As such, this review focuses primarily on the pathophysiology of atherosclerotic PAD.

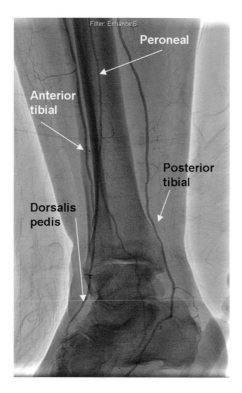

Figure 2.5

Angiogram of the tibial arteries and branches to the foot.

Table 2.1 Non-Atherosclerotic Causes of Peripheral Arterial Disease

Acute arterial disease (dissection, thrombosis, embolism)
Vasospasm (ergot toxicity, alpha-agonist toxicity)
Radiation fibrosis
Takayasu's arteritis
Thromboangiitis obliterans (Buerger's disease)
Adventitial cystic degeneration
Arterial aneurysm with thrombosis
Fibromuscular dysplasia
Pseudoxanthoma elasticum
Iliac endofibrosis (seen in endurance athletes/cyclists)
Popliteal artery entrapment syndrome
Compartment syndrome

Symptomatic peripheral arterial disease is caused by a disruption of the balance that normally exists between supply of nutrients to skeletal muscle and demand for these substances. This balance is typically lost in PAD when an arterial stenosis impedes adequate blood flow to skeletal muscle. As the vessel lumen narrows, a pressure gradient develops across the stenotic lesion proportional to blood viscosity and the length of the stenosis. The Poiseuille equation ($Q = \Delta P \pi r^4 / 8 \eta l$) describes the quantitative relationship between flow (Q) and the pressure gradient (ΔP), the radius of the lumen (r), blood viscosity (η), and the length of the affected stenotic vessel (l).

A stenosis that does not cause a pressure gradient at rest may result in a gradient when a second stenosis develops in series or when a patient exercises. During exercise, demand for skeletal muscle nutrients increases. In a normal individual during exercise, an increase in cardiac output and a decrease in systemic vascular resistance are sufficient to augment blood flow to skeletal muscle and compensate for the increased demand. However, an arterial stenosis that is not significant at rest may become apparent during exercise if increased peripheral muscle demands are not matched by augmented flow.

An important consideration in the pathophysiology of PAD is the significant functional impairment present in diseased peripheral arteries. This impairment manifests as diminished vasomotor function and enhanced vasoconstriction. Increased leukocyte adhesiveness, increased vascular and tissue level inflammation, increased platelet aggregation, and adverse muscle tissue characteristics have been noted in subjects with PAD and likely also contribute substantially to the genesis, progression, and symptomatology of PAD.

Atherosclerosis affects different segments of the arterial tree to varying degrees. This phenomenon is likely caused by a complex interplay of embryologic vascular origin and local environmental conditions. The embryologic origin of a vascular segment plays an important role in determining its morphology, physiology, and relative propensity for developing atherosclerosis. Local conditions, such as amount of shear stress, contribute to differential expression of transcriptional factors that can promote (or inhibit) atherogenesis. This helps to explain why some arterial segments, such as branch points, appear to have a greater likelihood of developing significant atherosclerotic disease.

EPIDEMIOLOGY/NATURAL HISTORY

The prevalence of PAD depends on the population studied and the diagnostic modality used to assess for disease. PAD, as defined by an ankle-brachial index (ABI) < 0.90 in either leg, is likely present in 4%–10% of patients in the United States and Europe.[1–4] PAD is thought to affect at least four to seven million people in the United States.

PAD dramatically increases in prevalence with advancing age, especially after age 40. In the National Health and Nutrition Evaluation Survey (NHANES), PAD was present in 0.9% of participants aged 40–49.[4] Among participants over age 70, by contrast, the prevalence of PAD increased to 14.5%.[2, 3] The highest prevalence of PAD noted to date was seen in participants in the Peripheral arterial disease Awareness, Risk and Treatment New Resources for Survival (PARTNERS) program, a study of almost 7,000 patients over age 70, or age 50–69 with diabetes or current smoking (> 10 pack-years). PAD was present in 29% of PARTNERS participants as assessed by history and ABI (Figure 2.6).[3]

Traditional cardiovascular risk factors appear to play a large role in the development of PAD. In general, PAD is more frequent in males, smokers, older age, and in patients with diabetes and hypertension.

The most important of these factors is cigarette smoking. In the Cardiovascular Health Study, the Framingham Study, and the NHANES studies, the risk of PAD was increased two to five times in active smokers.[4–6] Collectively, studies suggest that approximately 80% of patients with PAD are current or former smokers.[7, 8] Not only does smoking increase an individual's likelihood of developing PAD, it also appears to accelerate PAD progression. In the PARTNERS study, smokers aged 50–69 years had rates of PAD similar to those of non-smokers over 70.[3] Smoking cessation may only modestly decrease the risk of claudication: The Edinburgh Artery Study found that the relative risk of claudication decreased from 3.7 to 3 in patients who discontinued smoking for less than 5 years. It is unknown if the risk ever returns to baseline.[9]

In the Framingham Heart Study, the ratio of total-to-HDL cholesterol appeared to be the best lipid profile predictor of occurrence of PAD. Other factors that may play a

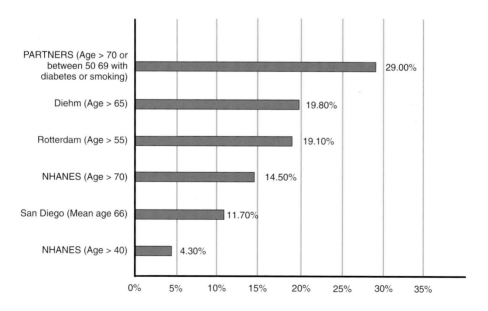

Figure 2.6

Prevalence of PAD in landmark trials. With information from references 1–4 and 7.

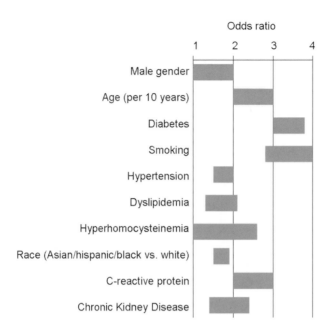

Figure 2.7

Approximate range of odds ratios for risk factors for symptomatic PAD.

Reprinted from: Eur J Vasc Endovasc Surg, Vol. 33, Suppl. 1, Norgren L, Hiatt WR, Dormandy JA, et al. Inter-Society Consensus for the Management of Peripheral Arterial Disease (TASC II), Pages S1–S75, Copyright, 2007, with permission from Elsevier.

role include hyperhomocysteinemia (detected in 30% of young patients with PAD) or chronic kidney disease.[10] Hyperviscosity, increased hematocrit (possibly from smoking), and hyperfibrinogenemia have been associated both as risk factors and as markers of poor prognosis in patients with PAD. Figure 2.7 shows an approximate range of odds ratios by risk factors for symptomatic PAD.

CLINICAL PRESENTATION

The ACC/AHA guidelines break down the spectrum of PAD into different categories:[11]

   i. Asymptomatic
  ii. Claudication
 iii. Critical limb ischemia
 iv. Acute limb ischemia

Figure 2.8 summarizes the morbidity and outcomes of patients with these clinical categories.

These clinical categories also have prognostic implications, as the survival of patients who develop intermittent claudication or critical limb ischemia is markedly lower than that of asymptomatic patients (Figures 2.9 and 2.10).

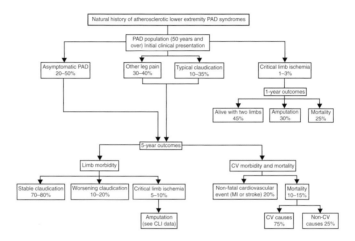

Figure 2.8

Clinical scenarios, morbidity and mortality of PAD. CLI, critical limb ischemia.

Reprinted from: Eur J Vasc Endovasc Surg, Vol. 33, Suppl. 1, Norgren L, Hiatt WR, Dormandy JA, et al. Inter-Society Consensus for the Management of Peripheral Arterial Disease (TASC II), Pages S1–S75, Copyright, 2007, with permission from Elsevier.

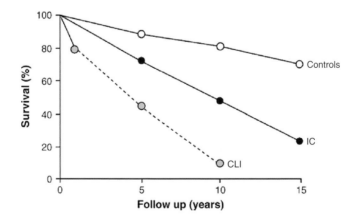

Figure 2.9

Survival of patients with peripheral arterial disease. IC, intermittent claudication; CLI, critical limb ischemia.

Reprinted from: Eur J Vasc Endovasc Surg, Vol. 33, Suppl. 1, Norgren L, Hiatt WR, Dormandy JA, et al. Inter-Society Consensus for the Management of Peripheral Arterial Disease (TASC II), Pages S1–S75, Copyright, 2007, with permission from Elsevier.

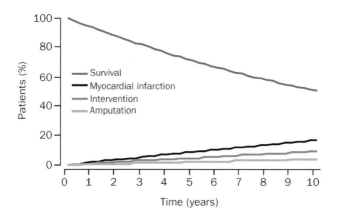

Figure 2.10

Survival, myocardial infarction, surgical or percutaneous revascularization, and major amputation over a 10-year follow-up in patients presenting initially with intermittent claudication.

Reprinted from: The Lancet, Vol. 358, Ouriel K. Peripheral arterial disease, Pages 1257–64, Copyright 2001, with permission from Elsevier.

Asymptomatic

Asymptomatic PAD has importance because there is evidence to suggest that the progression of the underlying PAD is identical, whether the patient experiences symptoms or not.[12] In addition, some asymptomatic patients may evolve to symptomatic disease, including critical limb ischemia, and may have other cardiovascular complications (Figure 2.8).

Fewer than 20% of patients with peripheral arterial disease report the typical symptom of intermittent claudication: exertional leg-muscle discomfort that is relieved with rest.[13]

Even when present, claudication is, by itself, poorly specific for PAD. In the Rotterdam Study, an ABI of less than 0.9 was found in only 69% of patients with claudication symptoms.[2] In contrast, in the Edinburgh Artery Study, 8% of asymptomatic patients had advanced PAD as determined by the World Health Organization questionnaire and ABI measurements.[9]

Patients with asymptomatic PAD usually have other cardiovascular risk factors. By identifying individuals with asymptomatic PAD, therapeutic interventions known to decrease their risk of PAD progression, MI, stroke, or death may be instituted.

Claudication

Claudication is defined as fatigue, discomfort, or pain that occurs in specific limb muscle groups during effort due to exercise-induced ischemia. The differential diagnosis of claudication includes the causes described in Table 2.2. Individuals with claudication have sufficient blood flow so that limb ischemic symptoms are absent at rest. With increased local muscular demand for metabolic support during exercise, blood flow in individuals with PAD and claudication is inadequate to meet this demand, and limb muscular fatigue or pain results.

Table 2.2   Causes of Lower Extremity Ischemia

Peripheral artery disease
Emboli
Radiation arteritis
Buerger's disease (thromboangiitis obliterans)
Other vasculitis or arteritis
Coarctation of the aorta (congenital or acquired)
Popliteal entrapment or aneurysm
Cystic adventitial disease
Fibromyalgia rheumatica
Trauma
Endofibrosis of the external iliac artery (iliac artery syndrome) in cyclists
Primary vascular tumors
Pseudoxanthoma elasticum

The anatomic site of the arterial stenosis is often associated with specific symptoms:

- Iliac artery stenosis may produce hip, buttock, thigh, and calf pain
- Femoral and popliteal stenosis is usually associated with calf pain
- Tibial artery stenosis may produce calf pain or, more rarely, foot pain and numbness

Table 2.3 provides insight into the differential diagnosis of claudication and pseudo-claudication (non-vascular pain).

Once the presence of claudication is documented, its severity may then be classified according to the Fontaine or the Rutherford categories (Table 2.4).

Critical Limb Ischemia

Unlike individuals with exertional claudication, patients with critical limb ischemia have inadequate perfusion at rest.

Critical limb ischemia is defined as extremity pain at rest or as impending limb loss that is caused by severe compromise of blood flow, including ulcers or gangrene attributable to PAD. The term critical limb ischemia implies chronicity and is to be distinguished from acute limb ischemia. If left untreated, it usually leads to major limb amputation within 6 months.

Although usually caused by atherosclerotic arterial disease, it can also be caused by atheroemboli, thromboemboli, vasculitis, hypercoagulable states, thromboangiitis obliterans, cystic adventitial disease, popliteal entrapment, or trauma.

Any factor that contributes to reduced blood flow to the microvasculature may exacerbate critical limb ischemia (e.g., low cardiac output, diabetes, vasospasm). In addition,

Table 2.3   Differential Diagnosis of Claudication and Pseudoclaudication

Condition	Location of Discomfort	Characteristic Discomfort	Onset Relative to Exercise	Walking Distance	Effect of Rest	Effect of Body Position	Other Characteristics
Calf intermittent claudication	Calf muscles	Cramping, aching discomfort. Also fatigue, weakness.	After same degree of exercise, no discomfort with standing	Reproducible	Quickly relieved	None	May have atypical limb symptoms on exercise. Reproducible, associated with atherosclerosis and decreased pulses.
Thigh and buttock intermittent claudication	Buttocks, hip, thigh	Cramping, aching discomfort. Also fatigue, weakness.	After same degree of exercise, no discomfort with standing	Reproducible	Quickly relieved	None	Erectile dysfunction. May have normal pulses with isolated iliac artery disease.
Foot intermittent claudication	Foot arch	Severe pain on exercise. Also fatigue, weakness.	After same degree of exercise, no discomfort with standing	Reproducible	Quickly relieved	None	May also present as numbness
Nerve root compression	Radiates down leg, usually posteriorly	Sharp lancinating pain	Soon, if not immediately relieved after onset. Induced by sitting, standing, or walking	Variable	Not quickly relieved (also often present at rest)	Relief may be aided by adjusting back position	History of back problems. Worse with sitting. Relief when supine or sitting.
Spinal stenosis	Hip, thigh, buttocks (follows dermatome)	Motor weakness more prominent than pain; tingling, weakness, clumsiness	After walking or standing for same length of time	Variable	Relieved by stopping only if position changed	Relief by lumbar spine flexion (sitting or stooping forward). Worse with standing and extending spine.	Frequent history of back problems, provoked by intra-abdominal pressure
Foot or ankle arthritis	Foot, arch	Aching pain	After variable degree of exercise	Variable	Not quickly relieved (may be present at rest)	May be relieved by not bearing weight	Variable, may relate to activity level; may be present at rest
Hip or knee arthritis	Hip, thigh, buttocks, knee	Aching discomfort, usually localized to hip and gluteal region or the knees	After variable degree of exercise or with standing	Variable	Not quickly relieved (may be present at rest)	More comfortable sitting, weight taken off legs (when not weight bearing)	Variable, may relate to activity level, weather changes, discomfort at joint spaces
Symptomatic Baker's cyst	Behind knee, down calf	Swelling, soreness, tenderness	With exercise	Variable	Present at rest	None	Not intermittent
Venous claudication	Entire leg, but usually worse in the calf	Tight, bursting pain	After walking, changes with shift in standing position	Variable	Subsides slowly	Relief speeded by elevation	History of iliofemoral deep vein thrombosis, signs of venous congestion, edema
Chronic compartment syndrome	Calf muscles	Tight, bursting pain	After much exercise (e.g., jogging); changes with shift in position	Variable	Subsides very slowly	Relief speeded by elevation	Typically heavy muscled athletes. May also present as numbness.

Adapted from references 11–14.

Table 2.4   Classification of Peripheral Arterial Disease: Fontaine's Stages and Rutherford's Categories

FONTAINE		RUTHERFORD		
Stage	Clinical	Grade	Category	Clinical
I	Asymptomatic	0	0	Asymptomatic
IIa	Mild claudication	I	1	Mild claudication
IIb	Moderate to severe claudication	I	2	Moderate claudication
		I	3	Severe claudication
III	Ischemic rest pain	II	4	Ischemic rest pain
IV	Ulceration or gangrene	III	5	Minor tissue loss
		III	6	Major tissue loss

Adapted from reference 12.

increase in the demand for blood supply may also exacerbate critical limb ischemia (e.g., infection, skin breakdown, trauma).

Patients with critical limb ischemia usually present with limb pain at rest and may have trophic skin changes or tissue loss. The discomfort is often worse when lying supine and may lessen when the limb is kept in the dependent position (Figures 2.11 and 2.12).

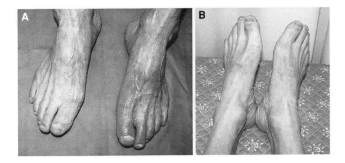

Figure 2.11

Photographs of common physical exam findings in a patient with claudication. In panel A, the left foot is erythematous, cold to touch, and pulseless in the dorsalis pedis and posterior tibial artery territories, while hanging down. In panel B, the foot becomes pale when the extremities are elevated. This is consistent with Buerger's sign, suggestive of peripheral artery disease. **See Plate 1 for color image.**

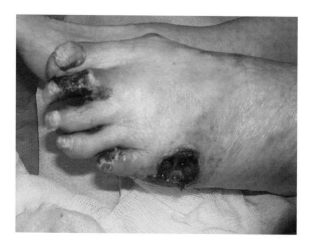

Figure 2.12

Critical limb ischemia. There is rubor of the forefoot, gangrene of the digits, and an ulceration. **See Plate 2 for color image.**

Reproduced with permission from the Cardiovascular and Interventional Radiological Society of Europe: http://www.cirse.org (accessed January, 2010).

When ulcers are the mode of presentation, it is sometimes difficult to differentiate between those caused by PAD and those caused by venous stasis or due to trauma in patients with neuropathy. Certain clues, however, can aid in the differential diagnosis of leg ulcers (Table 2.5).

Table 2.5   Differential Diagnosis of Common Foot and Leg Ulcers

ORIGIN	CAUSE	LOCATION	PAIN	APPEARANCE
Main arteries	Atherosclerotic lower extremity PAD, Buerger's disease, acute arterial occlusion	Toes, foot	Severe	Irregular, pink base
Venous	Venous disease	Malleolar	Mild	Irregular, pink base
Skin infarct	Systemic disease, embolism, hypertension	Lower third of leg	Severe	Small after infarction, often multiple
Neurotrophic	Neuropathy	Foot sole	None	Often deep, infected

Adapted from reference 11.

Acute Limb Ischemia

Acute limb ischemia is defined as a rapid or sudden decrease in limb perfusion that threatens tissue viability. It is a medical emergency. It may present either as progression of chronic ischemia or as a first manifestation in a previously asymptomatic patient.

Its severity depends on the location and extent of the arterial occlusion and the presence or absence of collaterals. It is also influenced by the peripheral vascular resistance and the cardiac output.

Acute limb ischemia is often associated with thrombosis due to plaque rupture, thrombosis of a lower extremity bypass graft, or lower extremity embolism originating from the heart or a proximal arterial aneurysm.

Traditionally, the physical exam reveals the 6 P's:

- Pain
- Paralysis
- Paresthesias
- Pulselessness (pulses may be normal in microembolism)
- Pallor
- Polar (cold)

Thrombosis due to plaque rupture occurs most frequently in the superficial femoral artery. The thrombus tends to propagate proximally and may compromise a more proximal branch.

Arterial embolism, in contrast, is suggested by:

- Sudden onset or sudden worsening of symptoms
- Known embolic source (atrial fibrillation, cardiomyopathy, left ventricular thrombus, atheromatous aorta, aortic or other arterial aneurysm, or, less commonly, paradoxical embolism through a patent foramen ovale).
- Absence of antecedent claudication
- Presence of normal pulses in the contralateral limb

Exceptions to the above signs are saddle embolism to the aortoiliac bifurcation and severe bilateral peripheral vascular disease.

Figure 2.13 provides estimates of the frequency by etiology of acute limb ischemia.

The differential diagnosis (Table 2.6) includes conditions that mimic atherosclerotic arterial occlusion (trauma, vasospasm, arteritis, hypercoagulable states, compartment syndrome, arterial dissection, external compression) or conditions that cause embolism (atrial fibrillation, left ventricular thrombus, paradoxical embolism).

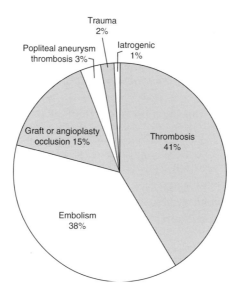

Figure 2.13

Etiology of acute limb ischemia.

Reprinted from: Eur J Vasc Endovasc Surg, Vol. 33, Suppl. 1, Norgren L, Hiatt WR, Dormandy JA, et al. Inter-Society Consensus for the Management of Peripheral Arterial Disease (TASC II), Pages S1–S75, Copyright, 2007, with permission from Elsevier.

Table 2.6   Differential Diagnosis of Acute Limb Ischemia

Conditions mimicking acute limb ischemia

- Systemic shock (especially if associated with chronic occlusive disease)
- Phlegmasia cerulea dolens (massive deep venous thrombosis)
- Acute compressive neuropathy

Differential diagnosis for acute limb ischemia (other than acute PAD)

- Arterial trauma
- Aortic/arterial dissection
- Arteritis with thrombosis (e.g., giant cell arteritis, thromboangiitis obliterans)
- HIV arteriopathy
- Spontaneous thrombosis associated with a hypercoagulable state
- Popliteal adventitial cyst with thrombosis
- Popliteal entrapment with thrombosis
- Vasospasm with thrombosis (e.g., ergotism)
- Compartment syndrome

Continues

Table 2.6   Differential Diagnosis of Acute Limb Ischemia (Continued)

Acute PAD

- Thrombosis of an atherosclerotic stenosed artery
- Thrombosis of an arterial bypass graft
- Embolism from heart, aneurysm, plaque, or critical stenosis upstream (including cholesterol or atherothrombotic emboli secondary to endovascular procedures)
- Thrombosed aneurysm with or without embolization

Table adapted from reference 12.

DIAGNOSTIC EVALUATION

Physical Exam

The physical exam should assess the circulatory system as a whole, including vital signs, blood pressure in both arms, and heart, neck, and abdominal exam. Vascular bruits, aneurysms, and skin or muscle atrophy should be sought.

The specific peripheral vascular examination requires palpation of the radial, ulnar, brachial, carotid, femoral, popliteal, dorsalis pedis, and posterior tibial artery pulses.

Palpation of peripheral pulses is subject to high interobserver variability but is the simplest way of evaluating for a peripheral artery stenosis or occlusion. Peripheral pulses should be graded as follows:

- 0 (absent)
- 1 (diminished)
- 2 (normal)

A recent systematic review of the physical exam diagnosis of PAD suggested that a scoring system for the physical exam, inclusive of auscultation of arterial components by handheld Doppler, provides greater diagnostic accuracy for PAD (Table 2.7).

Ankle Brachial Index

The ABI is the standard for the diagnosis of peripheral artery disease in the office, vascular laboratories, and epidemiological surveys. It is performed by measuring the systolic blood pressure from both brachial arteries and from both the dorsalis pedis and posterior tibial arteries after the patient has been in the supine position for 10 minutes (Figure 2.14). These recordings are obtained with appropriately sized cuffs, and systolic blood pressures are detected with a handheld 5 or 10 mHz Doppler. The systolic blood pressure difference between both arms should be less than 12 mmHg. If the difference is greater, it should raise suspicion for a subclavian or axillary arterial stenosis. The pulse wave reflection causes the ankle pressure to be 10 to 15 mmHg higher than that of the brachial artery. Therefore, a normal ABI should be greater than 1.00.

Table 2.7   Peripheral Artery Disease Score

DEFINITION		
Item	**Details**	**Score**
Number of *auscultated* components in the posterior tibial artery with handheld Doppler	Right + left posterior tibial artery	0 for none heard to 3 for normal for each artery
Plus		
Grade of *palpated* pulse in the posterior tibial artery	Right posterior tibial artery + left posterior tibial artery	2 for normal, 1 for palpated but abnormal, 0 for not palpable for each artery
Plus		
History	History of myocardial infarction	1 if no history 0 if prior myocardial infarction
	NORMAL SCORE	**LIKELIHOOD RATIO (LR) OF HAVING PAD**
Testing both legs	10	Score < 6, LR is 7.80 Score > 6, LR is 0.2
Testing one leg	5	Score < 4 LR is 5 Score > 4 LR is 0.1

Adapted from reference 15.

An ABI threshold of 0.90 has a sensitivity of 95% and a specificity of 100% when compared to angiography for the detection of PAD.[9] Values between 0.90 and 0.71 indicate mild obstruction, between 0.70 and 0.41 moderate obstruction, and less than 0.41 severe obstruction.

Falsely normal ABI values may be present in patients with severe iliofemoral artery stenosis or occlusion if sufficient collaterals are present, but are more likely in noncompressible vessels. Noncompressible vessels are present more frequently in patients with long-standing diabetes mellitus and advanced chronic kidney disease.

Noncompressible vessels should be suspected when the ABI is greater than 1.30 or when the systolic pressure in the lower extremities is greater than 20 mmHg or 20% higher than the brachial systolic pressure. In patients with noncompressible vessels, the toe-brachial index may be used. It is performed by placing a small occlusive cuff on the proximal portion of the great or second toe, with the return of toe pulsatility (representing systolic perfusion pressure) assessed by a plethysmograph. It is possible to obtain because the media of the digital arteries is usually spared from fibrosis and calcification.

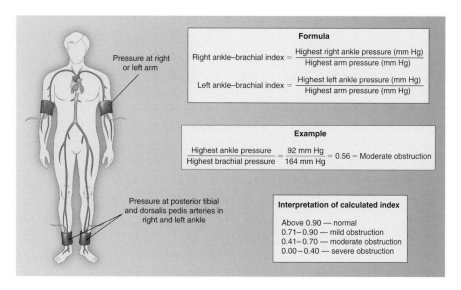

Figure 2.14

Performing pressure measurements and calculating the ankle-brachial index. To calculate the ankle-brachial index, systolic pressures are determined in both arms and both ankles with the use of a hand-held Doppler instrument. The highest readings for the dorsalis pedis and posterior tibial arteries are used to calculate the index.

ABI results have prognostic implications not only for progression of limb ischemia but also for cardiovascular events. The ABI is inversely related to the risk of myocardial infarction, stroke, or cardiovascular death (Figure 2.15).

Segmental Pressure Measurements and Pulse Volume Recording

It is possible to determine the location of individual arterial stenoses by placing blood pressure cuffs sequentially along the limb at various levels. A gradient of greater than 20 mmHg between adjacent segments is interpreted as a sign of a hemodynamically significant stenosis (Figure 2.16).

Arterial flow is pulsatile, and each pulse represents changes in volume, which can be measured by a plethysmographic device. Pulse volume recordings are a method of evaluating arterial pressure waveform profiles. Similar to segmental pressures, sequential cuffs are placed along the extremities. Its diagnostic accuracy is 90%–95%.[16] It is particularly useful to assess the severity of iliac and superficial femoral artery stenoses, but its accuracy decreases in distal segments.

Continuous-Wave Ultrasound

Continuous-wave ultrasound is helpful in assessing the location and severity of PAD, and in evaluating its progression. The pulsatility index is most commonly used as the parameter of reference. The pulsatility index is calculated as follows:

$$\text{Pulsatility Index} = \frac{\text{Peak systolic velocity} - \text{Minimum diastolic velocity}}{\text{Mean blood velocity}}$$

Normally, the pulsatility index increases from proximal to distal. A decrease in the pulsatility index between adjacent proximal and distal anatomic segments implies the presence of occlusive disease between these two locations. The degree of decline in the pulsatility index is proportional to the severity of the stenosis.

In addition to the pulsatility index, the analysis of the morphology of the Doppler waveform can add helpful information to localize the site of the stenosis.

Treadmill Exercise Testing with ABI

Treadmill exercise testing provides the most objective evidence of the degree of functional limitation, and permits assessment of response to therapy. In addition, by measurement

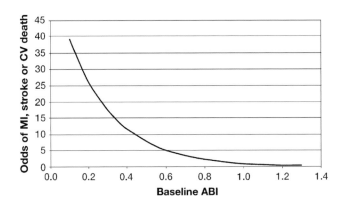

Figure 2.15

Adjusted odds of a cardiovascular event by ankle-brachial index. Some authors suggest that the distribution of events would probably have a J-shaped configuration with higher ABIs because mortality is also increased in patients with non-compressible vessels; however data is not available. ABI, ankle-brachial index; CV, cardiovascular; MI, myocardial infarction.

Reprinted from: Eur J Vasc Endovasc Surg, Vol. 33, Suppl. 1, Norgren L, Hiatt WR, Dormandy JA, et al. Inter-Society Consensus for the Management of Peripheral Arterial Disease (TASC II), Pages S1–S75, Copyright, 2007, with permission from Elsevier.

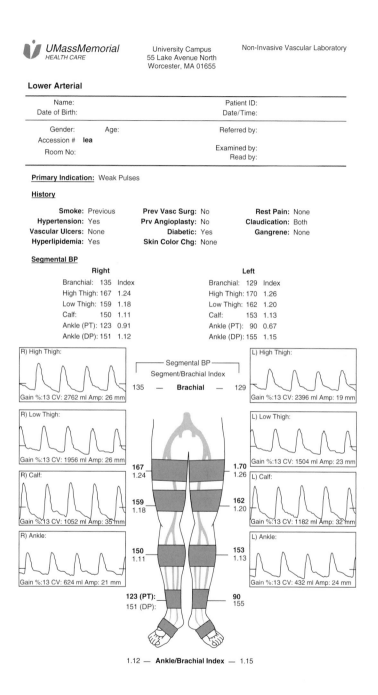

UMassMemorial
HEALTH CARE

University Campus
55 Lake Avenue North
Worcester, MA 01655

Non-Invasive Vascular Laboratory

Lower Arterial

Name: Patient ID:
Date of Birth: Date/Time:

Gender: Age: Referred by:
Accession #   **lea**
Room No: Examined by:
       Read by:

Primary Indication: Weak Pulses

History

Smoke: Previous	**Prev Vasc Surg:** No	**Rest Pain:** None
Hypertension: Yes	**Prv Angioplasty:** No	**Claudication:** Both
Vascular Ulcers: None	**Diabetic:** Yes	**Gangrene:** None
Hyperlipidemia: Yes	**Skin Color Chg:** None	

Segmental BP

Right			Left		
Branchial: 135	Index		Branchial: 129	Index	
High Thigh: 167	1.24		High Thigh: 170	1.26	
Low Thigh: 159	1.18		Low Thigh: 162	1.20	
Calf: 150	1.11		Calf: 153	1.13	
Ankle (PT): 123	0.91		Ankle (PT): 90	0.67	
Ankle (DP): 151	1.12		Ankle (DP): 155	1.15	

R) High Thigh:
Gain %:13 CV: 2762 ml Amp: 26 mm

Segmental BP
Segment/Brachial Index
135 — **Brachial** — 129

L) High Thigh:
Gain %:13 CV: 2396 ml Amp: 19 mm

R) Low Thigh:
Gain %:13 CV: 1956 ml Amp: 26 mm

L) Low Thigh:
Gain %:13 CV: 1504 ml Amp: 23 mm

167
1.24

1.70
1.26

R) Calf:
Gain %:13 CV: 1052 ml Amp: 35 mm

L) Calf:
Gain %:13 CV: 1182 ml Amp: 32 mm

159
1.18

162
1.20

R) Ankle:
Gain %:13 CV: 624 ml Amp: 21 mm

L) Ankle:
Gain %:13 CV: 432 ml Amp: 24 mm

150
1.11

153
1.13

123 (PT):
151 (DP):

90
155

1.12 — **Ankle/Brachial Index** — 1.15

Figure 2.16

Results of a normal segmental pressure and pulse volume recording.

of pre- and postexercise ABI, it is possible to differentiate between claudication and pseudoclaudication.

Vascular treadmill testing uses less intense workloads (e.g., Naughton, Gardner-Skinner, or Hiatt protocols) than those used in coronary disease testing (e.g., Bruce, modified Bruce protocols). Electrocardiographic recording during the vascular treadmill test may provide evidence of inducible ischemia, but heart rate or workload are not considered test endpoints. Vascular treadmill testing is symptom (or protocol-completion) limited. Patients are instructed to indicate any symptoms. The test is stopped when mandated by symptoms, completion of protocol, significant ST depressions, or if arrhythmias ensue. After completing the test, the patient is placed in the supine position and both the brachial and the ankle pressures are recorded at 1 minute intervals until they reach the pre-exercise baseline.

An alternative to treadmill exercise is a 6-minute walk test, which is particularly helpful in the elderly or those not amenable to perform treadmill testing. In this test, the patients are asked to ambulate down corridors for a maximum of 6 minutes.

The pedal plantar flexion test is an option if a treadmill is not available. In this test, individuals with suspected PAD but normal ABI at rest are asked to stand flat-footed and perform 50 sequential, symptom-limited ankle plantar flexions and thus raise the heels maximally off the floor. Postexercise ABI values measured with this test are similar to those recorded in treadmill exercise.[17]

Duplex Ultrasound

Duplex ultrasound (Figure 2.17) is useful in the diagnosis of the location and the severity of PAD. It is also very useful in evaluating aneurysms, arterial dissections, popliteal artery entrapment syndrome, evaluation of lymphoceles, and assessment of soft tissue masses.

Duplex ultrasound provides images in two dimensions and with color Doppler, but quantitative criteria are based on spectral Doppler velocities. The most commonly used quantitative criterion is the peak systolic velocity ratio (a ratio > 2 is found in stenoses > 50%, with a sensitivity and specificity of 90% and 95%, respectively).[11]

Duplex ultrasound is also recommended for routine surveillance after femoral-popliteal or femoral-tibial/pedal bypass with venous conduits. The detection of stenoses in venous conduits should prompt consideration for graft revision, regardless of symptoms or ABI. This aggressive approach has been associated with increased graft patency.[18] The recommended surveillance intervals are 3, 6, and 12 months and annually thereafter.[11]

The value of Duplex ultrasound in the surveillance of synthetic grafts or after angioplasty is questionable and is not recommended.

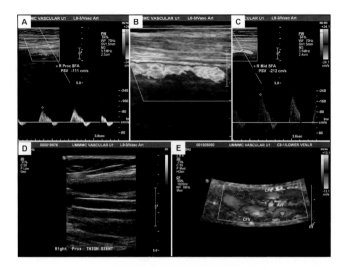

Figure 2.17

Duplex ultrasound of the lower extremities. Panels A to C: Normal velocity in the superficial femoral artery (Panel A) proximal to a stenosis that produces color aliasing due to turbulent flow (Panel B) and an intra- and post-stenotic increase in flow velocity distal to the stenosis (Panel C). Panel D: Two-dimensional ultrasound of a patent superficial femoral artery stent. Panel E: Iatrogenic arteriovenous fistula (AVF, arteriovenous fistula; CFA, common femoral artery; CFV, common femoral vein; arrow indicates the fistulous communication). **See Plate 3 for color image.**

Images courtesy of Denise Kush, RDMS, RVT; Vascular Laboratory, UMass Memorial Health Care.

Figure 2.18 presents an algorithm with different methods and diagnostic criteria for the diagnosis of PAD in the vascular laboratory.

Computed Tomographic Angiography

Computed tomographic angiography (CTA) may be considered to diagnose the anatomic location and presence of significant stenoses in patients with PAD (Figure 2.19). It involves exposure to ionizing radiation and the administration of intravascular contrast media (approximately 100 to 180 cc). Advantages of multidetector CTA include the possibility of image reconstruction that allows rotation in every angle to evaluate eccentric stenoses, as well as three-dimensional reconstruction. It also visualizes the surrounding tissues, permitting differentiation between PAD and other entities causing extrinsic vascular compression. Its sensitivity and specificity to detect stenoses > 50% have been as high as 95% and 100%, respectively. It has certain advantages over other diagnostic tests, like magnetic resonance angiography, as CTA can be safely performed in patients with pacemakers and surgical metallic clips. Calcium quantification is also possible with CTA.[11, 12]

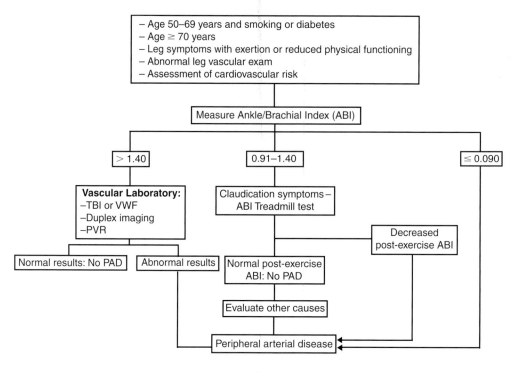

Figure 2.18

Algorithm for the diagnosis of PAD in the vascular laboratory. TBI, toe-brachial index; VWF, velocity wave form; PVR, pulse volume recording.

Reprinted from: Eur J Vasc Endovasc Surg, Vol. 33, Suppl. 1, Norgren L, Hiatt WR, Dormandy JA, et al. Inter-Society Consensus for the Management of Peripheral Arterial Disease (TASC II), Pages S1–S75, Copyright, 2007, with permission from Elsevier.

CTA has proven to be a useful tool in the surveillance of patients with grafts when physical exam or Duplex evaluations are abnormal. It can be used to detect:[19]

- New stenotic lesions
- Anastomotic stenoses
- Aneurysmal degenerations
- Local complications (hemorrhage, graft thrombosis, infection)

Magnetic Resonance Angiography

Magnetic resonance angiography (MRA) is useful to diagnose the location and severity of stenotic lesions (Figure 2.20). It should be performed with gadolinium enhancement. There are multiple MRA techniques, each with its own advantages and disadvantages.

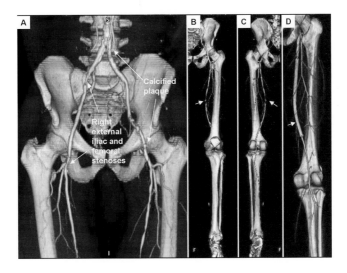

Figure 2.19

Computed tomography angiography of the iliac and lower extremity vessels. Panel A: Three-dimensional CTA reconstruction revealing calcified plaque and stenoses of the right external iliac and right femoral arteries. Panel B: Anterior view of a three-dimensional CTA reconstruction in a patient with significant superficial femoral artery stenosis (arrow). Panel C: Posterior view of a three-dimensional CTA reconstruction in a patient with significant superficial femoral artery stenosis (arrow). Panel D: Posterior view of a three-dimensional CTA reconstruction in a patient with a superficial femoral artery stent (arrow).

Figures courtesy of David J. Sheehan, DO; Radiology Department, University of Massachusetts Medical Center and Medical School.

Techniques and protocols include two-dimensional time of flight, three-dimensional imaging, contrast enhancement with gadolinium, substraction, cardiac gating, and bolus chase. These can be used alone or in combination. The sensitivity and specificity of MRA for detection of stenoses > 50% are both in the range of 95%–100%, with greater accuracy when gadolinium is used.[20]

MRA has certain limitations: It tends to overestimate the degree of stenosis due to turbulence. In addition, certain metal stents may obscure vascular flow visualization, and metal clips can cause artifacts that mimic vessel occlusions. Patients with pacemakers, defibrillators, and certain brain aneurysm clips cannot be scanned. Gadolinium has also been associated with the development of nephrogenic systemic fibrosis. Ten percent of patients may not be able to tolerate MRA due to claustrophobia.

MRA may be considered for assessment of graft patency. When evaluating vein grafts, it has a sensitivity and specificity of 90% and 98.3%, respectively.[21] However, there are no studies showing improved outcomes from revascularization based on MRA surveillance.[11]

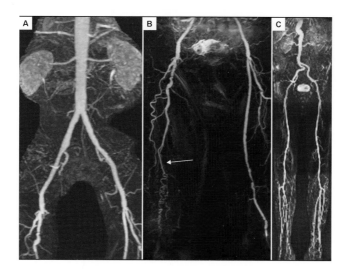

Figure 2.20

Magnetic resonance angiography of the lower extremity circulation. Panel A: The aortoiliac and iliofemoral circulation. Panel B: Iliofemoral tree; total occlusion of the superficial femoral artery with collateral flow (arrow). Panel C: Distal runoff.

Figures A and B courtesy of David J. Sheehan, DO; Radiology Department, University of Massachusetts Medical Center and Medical School. Figure C courtesy of Raul Galvez, MD, MPH and Hale Ersoy, MD; Radiology Department, Brigham and Women's Hospital, Harvard Medical School.

Contrast Angiography

Angiography is the gold standard for the anatomic evaluation of patients with PAD. Digital subtraction angiography (DSA), which digitally removes artifact caused by bone and other tissues, is the preferred method, as it allows for enhanced imaging capabilities when compared to conventional angiography.

It entails exposure to ionizing radiation, the administration of intravascular contrast media, and is an invasive procedure with its own associated risks (atheroembolization, dissection, vessel perforation, bleeding, etc.).

Many centers obtain detailed DSA for intervention planning, while others rely on non-invasive tests for general assessment and intervention planning, and use supraselective DSA immediately prior to the intervention. Advantages of the latter approach are better image definition and smaller doses of contrast.

Other diagnostic methods may be superior to angiography in certain situations, e.g., critical limb ischemia with poor inflow to the leg and below-knee vessels that are difficult to identify by DSA.

Angiography is used to guide percutaneous peripheral interventional procedures. These include functional assessments of stenotic lesions by pressure gradients, intravascular ultrasound, angioscopy, etc., as well as percutaneous revascularization.

Table 2.8 summarizes advantages and disadvantages of different imaging modalities.

Evaluation in Other Clinical Categories

Asymptomatic PAD

Current guidelines recommend screening for asymptomatic PAD as follows:[11]

- Patients > 70 years of age
- Patients between ages 50 and 70 and cardiovascular risk factors
- Patients of age < 50 with diabetes and cardiovascular risk factors

Screening should be performed as follows:

- Review of systems inclusive of walking impairment, claudication, ischemic rest pain, non-healing wounds
- Measurement of the ABI

The use of questionnaires alone tends to underestimate the presence of leg symptoms, whereas physical examination of the pulses has a high interobserver variability and poor sensitivity. These are reasons why ABI measurement is helpful in establishing the diagnosis of PAD.

ABI measurement not only identifies individuals with asymptomatic PAD but also is associated with prognosis, as the risk of progression to limb-threatening ischemia increases by 20%–25% for each 0.1-unit decrease in the ABI.[22, 23]

Critical limb ischemia

The evaluation of patients with critical limb ischemia should consider:

- Confirmation of the diagnosis
- Localization of the lesion
- Assessment of the requirements for successful revascularization
- Assessment of the endovascular or operative risk

Patients with critical limb ischemia should undergo a comprehensive evaluation, acknowledging their very high risk for cardiovascular morbidity and mortality.

- Clinical history and examination, including the coronary and cerebral circulation
- Hematologic and biochemical tests: Complete blood count, platelet count, fasting blood glucose, hemoglobin

Table 2.8   Comparison of Different Imaging Methods

Modality	Availability	Relative Risk and Complications	Strengths	Weaknesses	Contraindications
X-ray contrast angiography	Widespread	High Access-site complications; contrast nephropathy; radiation exposure	"Established modality"	2D images, limited planes; imaging pedal vessels and collaterals in the setting of occlusion requires prolonged imaging and substantial radiation	Chronic kidney disease; contrast allergy
Multidetector computed tomography angiography	Moderate	Moderate Contrast nephropathy; radiation exposure	Rapid imaging; sub-millimeter voxel resolution; 3D volumetric information from axial slices; plaque morphology	Calcium causes "blooming artifact"; stented segments difficult to visualize	Chronic kidney disease; contrast allergy
Magnetic resonance angiography	Moderate	None	True 3D imaging modality; infinite planes and orientations can be constructed; plaque morphology from proximal segments with additional seque-nces; calcium does not cause artifact	Stents cause artifact, but alloys such as nitinol produce minimal artifact	Intracranial devices, spinal stimulators, pace-makers, cochlear implants, and intracranial clips and shunts are absolute contraindications
Duplex	Widespread	None	Hemodynamic information	Operator dependent and time consuming to image both lower extremities; calcified segments are difficult to assess	None

Table adapted from TASC II.[12]

- Hemoglobin A1C, creatinine, fasting lipid profile, and urinalysis (for glycosuria and proteinuria)
- Resting electrocardiogram
- Ankle or toe pressure measurement or other objective measures for the severity of ischemia
- Imaging of the lower limb arteries in patients considered for endovascular or surgical intervention
- Duplex scan of the carotid arteries should be considered in selected patients at high risk (defined as individuals with cerebrovascular ischemic symptoms or in whom the risk of carotid revascularization is less than the short-term risk of stroke)
- A more detailed coronary assessment may be performed in selected patients in whom coronary ischemic symptoms would otherwise merit such an assessment regardless of the presence of critical limb ischemia

THERAPEUTIC CONSIDERATIONS

Medical Treatment of Claudication

Figure 2.21 is an algorithm with general considerations for the medical treatment of PAD.

Supervised exercise programs

Current guidelines consider supervised exercise programs as a primary and efficacious treatment modality in patients with claudication. It achieves greater increases in maximal walking ability than drug therapies. Regular walking in a supervised claudication exercise program is expected to result in an increase in the speed and distance walked, with a decrease in claudication symptoms. This is achieved because exercise alters skeletal muscle metabolism, improves endothelial function, and promotes angiogenesis.[24, 25]

Supervised exercise programs are expected to provide functional benefits as early as 4 weeks after initiating therapy, but its effects are more evident after at least 12 weeks of therapy. Exercise is better when each session lasts longer than 30 minutes, if exercise takes place at least three times a week, when patients ambulate to near-maximal pain and when the program lasts 6 months or longer. Exercise can improve walking distance by 150%.[26, 27]

Exercise should take place initially three times a week, beginning with 30 minutes of training, but then increasing to 1 hour per session. During the exercise session, treadmill exercise is performed at a speed and grade that will induce claudication. It is important for the patient to stop when this claudication is considered moderate (stopping at the

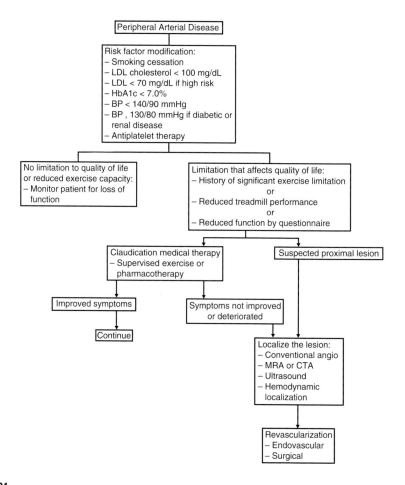

Figure 2.21

Overall treatment strategy for PAD. BP, blood pressure; HbA1c, hemoglobin A1c; LDL, low density lipoprotein.

Reprinted from: Eur J Vasc Endovasc Surg, Vol. 33, Suppl. 1, Norgren L, Hiatt WR, Dormandy JA, et al. Inter-Society Consensus for the Management of Peripheral Arterial Disease (TASC II), Pages S1–S75, Copyright, 2007, with permission from Elsevier.

onset of claudication is considered inadequate). The patient should then rest until the symptoms resolve, and ambulation is then resumed.

In a recent randomized trial of 156 patients with PAD, with and without claudication, supervised treadmill training improved 6-minute walk performance, treadmill walking performance, brachial artery flow-mediated dilation, and quality of life. In addition, lower extremity resistance training improved functional performance measured by treadmill walking, quality of life, and stair-climbing ability.[28]

Table 2.9 provides general guidelines for exercise training programs.

Table 2.9 Key Elements of a Therapeutic Claudication Exercise Training Program (PAD Rehabilitation)

Primary clinician role

- Establish the PAD diagnosis
- Determine that claudication is the major symptom limiting exercise
- Discuss risk/benefit of claudication therapeutic alternatives, including pharmacological, percutaneous, and surgical interventions
- Initiate systemic atherosclerosis risk modification
- Perform treadmill stress testing
- Provide formal referral to a claudication exercise rehabilitation program

Exercise guidelines for claudication

- Warm-up and cool-down period of 5 to 10 minutes each
- Types of exercise
  - Treadmill and track walking are the most effective exercise for claudication
  - Resistance training has conferred benefit to individuals with other forms of cardiovascular disease, and its use, as tolerated, for general fitness is complementary to but not a substitute for walking
- Intensity
  - The initial workload of the treadmill is set to a speed and grade that elicit claudication symptoms within 3 to 5 minutes
  - Patients walk at this workload until they achieve claudication of moderate severity, which is then followed by a brief period of standing or sitting rest to permit symptoms to resolve
- Duration
  - The exercise-rest-exercise pattern should be repeated throughout the exercise session
  - The initial duration will usually include 35 minutes of intermittent walking and should be increased by 5 minutes each session until 50 minutes of intermittent walking can be accomplished
- Frequency
  - Treadmill or track walking 3 to 5 times per week

Role of direct supervision

- As patients improve their walking ability, the exercise workload should be increased by modifying the treadmill grade or speed (or both) to ensure that there is always the stimulus of claudication pain during the workout
- As patients increase their walking ability, there is the possibility that cardiac signs and symptoms may appear (e.g., dysrhythmia, angina, or ST-segment depression). These events should prompt physician re-evaluation

Table adapted from reference 11.

Cilostazol

Cilostazol is a phosphodiesterase inhibitor that increases cAMP. It has vasodilator and antiplatelet properties. Seven randomized trials have found that cilostazol improves maximal walking distance by 40%–60% when compared to placebo. It also improves quality of life. A dose of 100 mg twice daily appears to be most effective.[29]

Its most common side effects include headache, diarrhea, palpitations, and dizziness. It should not be administered to patients with heart failure, as other phosphodiesterase inhibitors have been associated with increased mortality in patients with heart failure, with decreased ejection fraction.

Antiplatelet and anticoagulant agents

Antiplatelet therapy is indicated to reduce the risk of MI, stroke, or vascular death in patients with PAD.

The Antithrombotic Trialists' Collaboration performed a meta-analysis of 135,000 patients with previous MI, stroke, or PAD treated with aspirin. There was a 22% odds reduction of MI, stroke, or vascular death. In that meta-analysis, there was a 23% reduction of vascular events in patients with intermittent claudication, a 22% reduction in those with peripheral arterial grafts, and a 29% decrease in those undergoing angioplasty.[30]

With different doses of aspirin, the proportional reduction in vascular events was 32% with 75–150 mg daily, 26% with 160–325 mg daily, and 19% with 500–1500 mg daily.[30]

Antiplatelet therapy may also reduce the risk of progression to arterial occlusion in patients with PAD (by 20% over a 19-month period in one study).[31] A meta-analysis of 54 randomized, controlled trials in patients with intermittent claudication found that aspirin compared with placebo reduced the risk of arterial occlusion, and ticlopidine reduced the need for revascularization procedures.[32]

Dual antiplatelet therapy does not appear to have a role in the primary prevention of cardiovascular events: The CHARISMA trial evaluated 15,603 patients with either clinically evident cardiovascular disease or multiple risk factors to receive low-dose aspirin plus placebo or clopidogrel. The primary endpoint was a composite of myocardial infarction, stroke, or death from cardiovascular causes. There were no significant differences, with a trend of benefit in patients with symptomatic atherothrombosis, and a trend of harm in patients with only risk factors and no clinical cardiovascular disease. Interestingly, a secondary endpoint included the first occurrence of the composite endpoint plus hospitalization for unstable angina, transient ischemic attack, or revascularization (including peripheral). The incidence of this composite secondary endpoint was 11.1% in the ASA + clopidogrel vs. 12.3% in the ASA + placebo group, relative risk 0.9 (0.82–0.98), p = 0.02. The absolute risk reduction was only 1.2% in favor of dual antiplatelet therapy, but this group also had an increase in moderate bleeding, defined as hemodynamically stable bleeding requiring a blood transfusion.[33]

There is no role for long-term anticoagulation to increase infrainguinal graft patency. One trial randomized patients to ASA 81 mg daily or to coumadin with a target INR of 3 to 4.5. There were a similar number of graft occlusions and a significant increase in major bleeding in patients who were randomized to coumadin.[34] Other trials using lesser intensity regimens of anticoagulation did not affect rates of graft patency and were also associated with significant bleeding. Oral anticoagulants should, therefore, be limited to patients with other clinical indications for these agents.

The role of anticoagulation for the prevention of cardiovascular events in patients with PAD is controversial. A recent randomized trial with 2,000 patients with PAD, assigned to antiplatelet agents plus oral anticoagulants to a target INR of 2 to 3 versus antiplatelet agents alone did not show a reduction of myocardial infarction, stroke, and death from cardiovascular causes in this population. Furthermore, life-threatening bleeding occurred more frequently in the combination therapy group (4% vs. 1.2%, relative risk 3.41).[35] This is in contrast with a previous meta-analysis of 7 trials of moderate-intensity oral antico-agulation plus aspirin versus aspirin alone to prevent cardiovascular events in patients with coronary artery disease, which found a 12% odds reduction in cardiovascular death, MI, and stroke in favor of combined therapy.[36]

In summary, antiplatelet agents reduce overall cardiovascular mortality and may reduce the risk of progression to arterial occlusion. Anticoagulation has not proven to be effective in reducing cardiovascular events or PAD progression in patients with PAD.

Antihypertensive drugs
Treatment of hypertension is indicated to reduce the risk of cardiovascular events. The Joint National Committee-7 guidelines recommend a goal blood pressure of less than 140/90 mmHg for most patients, and less than 130/80 mmHg in patients with chronic kidney disease or with diabetes.[37]

In the past, concern had been expressed regarding the use of beta-blockers in patients with PAD, as they could theoretically worsen peripheral vasoconstriction by unopposed alpha-receptor agonism. A meta-analysis with 11 placebo-controlled trials in patients with intermittent claudication found that beta-blockers did not affect walking capacity.[38] Current guidelines clearly state that beta-blockers are not contraindicated in patients with PAD.[11]

Another indication for antihypertensive agents may not be blood pressure itself, but rather improvement in endothelial function and reduction of cardiovascular mortality. This is derived from the Heart Outcomes Prevention Evaluation (HOPE) study, which randomized patients with CAD, cerebrovascular disease, PAD, or diabetes to ramipril or placebo. Ramipril reduced the risk of MI, stroke, or vascular death in patients with PAD by approximately 25%. It is recommended that ACE inhibitors be considered as treatment for patients with both symptomatic and asymptomatic lower extremity PAD to reduce the risk of adverse cardiovascular events.[39]

Lipid-lowering agents
Patients with PAD are at the highest risk for cardiovascular events. Treatment of dyslipi-demia reduces the risk of adverse cardiovascular events in patients with atherosclerosis. The Heart Protection Study randomized patients with CAD, cerebrovascular disease, PAD,

or diabetes and a total cholesterol greater than 135 mg/dL to simvastatin or placebo. There was a 25% risk reduction in major adverse cardiac events at 5 years of follow-up.[40]

Patients with PAD should be treated to a goal LDL cholesterol of less than 100 mg/dL, and evidence suggests that less than 70 mg/dL may be better. Once the LDL goal is reached, other targets include lowering the non-HDL cholesterol to less than 130 mg/dL and to increase the HDL cholesterol to more than 40 mg/dL.[11, 12, 41]

In addition to lowering cardiovascular mortality, statins may also improve symptoms of intermittent claudication and walking distance.[42, 43]

Niacin and binding resins have been shown to reduce the progression of femoral artery atherosclerosis. They also appear to decrease cardiovascular events in patients with coronary artery disease.[44-46]

The role of fibrates in PAD has not been well established.[11]

Treatment of diabetes

It is not known if aggressive treatment of diabetes decreases the risk of peripheral vascular events in patients with PAD. In the Diabetes Control and Complications Trial (DCCT),[50] there was a non-significant reduction of claudication, peripheral revascularization, or amputation in patients with type 1 diabetes and intensive insulin therapy. The UK Prospective Diabetes Study (UKPDS)[51] did not show a reduction in the risk of amputations in patients with type 2 diabetes who had more aggressive glucose control. These trials, however, showed a marked reduction in major cardiovascular events, and optimal management of diabetes is advocated based on this risk reduction.[47, 48] Similarly, the prospective pioglitazone clinical trial in macrovascular events (PROACTIVE) study showed that pioglitazone decreased all-cause mortality, non-fatal myocardial infarction, and stroke in high-risk type 2 diabetes patients; however, there was no statistically significant difference in leg amputation or leg revascularization.[49]

Smoking cessation

Observational data have shown that the risk of death, MI, or amputation is substantially greater in patients who smoke than in those who stop smoking. Smoking cessation may also be associated with increased exercise time. Patients with PAD who smoke or use other forms of tobacco should be advised to stop smoking and should be offered comprehensive smoking cessation interventions, including behavioral therapy, nicotine replacement therapy, or other medications (e.g., Bupropion, Varenicline).[11]

Naftidrofuryl

This medication is only available in Europe. Naftidrofuryl is a 5-hydroxytryptamine type 2 antagonist that may improve muscle metabolism and reduce erythrocyte and platelet aggregation. In a meta-analysis of five studies involving a total of 888 patients, this medication increased pain-free walking distance by 26%.[50] Other studies have shown similar results on treadmill performance. The usual dose is 600 mg/day.

Carnitine

Propionyl-L-carnitine was shown to improve walking distance and quality of life in two multicenter trials with nearly 700 patients.[51, 52] Propionyl-L-carnitine is probably more effective than L-carnitine. These medications exert their effects by interacting with the skeletal muscle oxidative metabolism.

Other treatments

Pentoxifylline may be considered as a second-line alternative therapy to cilostazol to improve walking distance in patients with intermittent claudication. It has been associated with marginal but statistically significant improvement in pain-free and maximal walking distance. Its dose is 400 mg PO three times a day, requiring renal dose adjustments.[53]

Isovolemic hemodilution was used historically for the treatment of claudication, probably by reducing blood viscosity. It is only of historical interest.

Vasodilators have not been shown to have clinical efficacy in randomized controlled trials, although contemporary data are not available.[54] This applies to drugs that inhibit the sympathetic nervous system (alpha-blockers), direct-acting vasodilators (papaverine), beta2-adrenergic agonists (nylidrin), calcium channel blockers (nifedipine) and angiotensin-converting enzyme inhibitors (although in the HOPE trial, ACE inhibitors decreased cardiovascular events).[39] It has been hypothesized that these drugs may create a steal phenomenon by dilating vessels in normally perfused tissues, shifting the distribution of blood flow away from muscles supplied by obstructed arteries.

Other drugs with insufficient evidence of clinical utility include L-arginine, Acyl coenzyme A-cholesterol acyltransferase inhibitors, 5-hydroxytryptamine antagonists, prostaglandins, the vasodilator buflomedil, the hemorrheological Defibrotide, vitamin E, chelation therapy, omega-3 fatty acids, gingko biloba, and homocysteine-lowering drugs (vitamin B12 and folic acid).[11, 12]

Basic fibroblast growth factor (bFGF) stimulates the development of new vessels. It has been shown to improve exercise performance when given intra-arterially to patients with claudication.[55] The intramuscular administration of vascular endothelial growth factor (VEGF) has been shown to induce therapeutic angiogenesis in animal models and in selected patients with critical limb ischemia.[56]

Interventional Treatment of Claudication

Interventional approaches may have a significant impact on patients' symptom control and quality of life. Table 2.10 summarizes the indications for revascularization in patients with intermittent claudication.

Patients selected for possible revascularization may undergo additional imaging studies to determine whether their arterial anatomy is suitable for percutaneous or for surgical revascularization.

To understand the different interventional approaches, either percutaneous or surgical, it is necessary to first differentiate between different types of lesions, both anatomically and morphologically.

The TransAtlantic Inter-Society Consensus II (TASC) II guidelines simplify this by separating two anatomically different types of disease (Tables 2.11 and 2.12; Figures 2.22 through 2.25):

- Iliac lesions
- Femoropopliteal lesions

These are further stratified depending on the morphology, specific location, and length of the stenotic lesion.

Table 2.10   Indications for Revascularization in Intermittent Claudication

Before a patient with intermittent claudication is offered the option of any invasive revascularization therapy, whether endovascular or surgical, the following considerations must be taken into account:

- a predicted or observed lack of adequate response to exercise therapy and claudication pharmacotherapies
- the presence of a severe disability, with the patient either being unable to perform normal work or having very serious impairment of other activities important to the patient
- absence of other disease that would limit exercise even if the claudication was improved (e.g., angina or chronic respiratory disease)
- the anticipated natural history and prognosis of the patient
- the morphology of the lesion, which must be such that the appropriate intervention would have low risk and a high probability of initial and long-term success

Table adapted from reference 11.

Table 2.11   Morphological Stratification of Iliac Lesions

Type of Lesion	Preferred Treatment
TASC type A iliac lesions: • Single stenosis less than 3 cm of the CIA or EIA (unilateral/bilateral)	Endovascular
TASC type B iliac lesions: • Single stenosis 3 to 10 cm in length, not extending into the CFA • Total of two stenoses less than 5 cm long in the CIA and/or EIA and not extending into the CFA • Unilateral CIA occlusion	Either endovascular or surgical

TASC type C iliac lesions:	Either endovascular or surgical
• Bilateral 5- to 10-cm-long stenosis of the CIA and/or EIA, not extending into the CFA • Unilateral EIA occlusion not extending into the CFA • Unilateral EIA stenosis extending into the CFA • Bilateral CIA occlusion	
TASC type D iliac lesions:	Surgery
• Diffuse, multiple unilateral stenoses involving the CIA, EIA, and CFA (usually more than 10 cm long) • Unilateral occlusion involving both the CIA and EIA • Bilateral EIA occlusions • Diffuse disease involving the aorta and both iliac arteriesIliac stenoses in a patient with an abdominal aortic aneurysm or other lesion requiring aortic or iliac surgery	

Key: CFA, common femoral artery; CIA, common iliac artery; EIA, external iliac artery; TASC, TransAtlantic Inter-Society Consensus. Adapted from reference 11.

Table 2.12 Morphological Stratification of Femoropopliteal Lesions

TYPE OF LESION	TREATMENT OF CHOICE
TASC type A femoropopliteal lesions: • Single stenosis less than 3 cm of the superficial femoral artery or popliteal artery	Endovascular
TASC type B femoropopliteal lesions: • Single stenosis 3 to 10 cm in length, not involving the distal popliteal artery • Heavily calcified stenoses up to 3 cm in length • Multiple lesions, each less than 3 cm (stenoses or occlusions) • Single or multiple lesions in the absence of continuous tibial runoff to improve inflow for distal surgical bypass	More evidence needed
TASC type C femoropopliteal lesions: • Single stenosis or occlusion longer than 5 cm • Multiple stenoses or occlusions, each 3 to 5 cm in length, with or without heavy calcification	More evidence needed
TASC type D femoropopliteal lesions: • Complete common femoral artery or superficial femoral artery occlusions or complete popliteal and proximal trifurcation occlusions	Surgery

Table adapted from reference 11.

Type A lesions

- Unilateral or bilateral stenoses of CIA
- Unilateral or bilateral single short (≤3 cm) stenosis of EIA

Type B lesions

- Short (≤3 cm) stenosis of infrarenal aorta
- Unilateral CIA occlusion
- Single or multiple stenosis totaling 3–10 cm involving the EIA not extending into the CFA
- Unilateral EIA occlusion not involving the origins of internal iliac or CFA

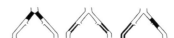

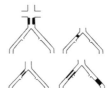

Type C lesions

- Bilateral CIA occlusions
- Bilateral EIA stenoses 3–10 cm long not extending into the CFA
- Unilateral EIA stenosis extending into the CFA
- Unilateral EIA occlusion that involves the origins of internal iliac and/or CFA
- Heavily calcified unilateral EIA occlusion with or without involvement of origins of internal iliac and/or CFA

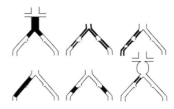

Type D lesions

- Infrarenal aortoiliac occlusion
- Diffuse disease involving the aorta and both iliac arteries requiring treatment
- Diffuse multiple stenoses involving the unilateral CIA, EIA, and CFA
- Unilateral occlusions of both CIA and EIA
- Bilateral occlusions of EIA
- Iliac stenoses in patients with AAA requiring treatment and not amenable to endograft placement or other lesions requiring open aortic or iliac surgery

Figure 2.22

Summary of preferred options for interventional management of iliac lesions.

Reprinted from: J Vasc Surg, Vol. 3, Dormandy JA, Rutherford RB. Management of peripheral arterial disease. TASC working group, Pages S1-S296. Copyright, 2000, with permission from Elsevier.

Surgical procedures are classified depending on three major patterns of arterial obstruction:

a. Inflow disease (suprainguinal vessels: Infrarenal aorta and iliac arteries). Typically presenting with buttock and thigh claudication or erectile dysfunction. Symptoms may progress to calf claudication.

b. Outflow disease (infrainguinal vessels: From the common femoral artery to the infrapopliteal trifurcation). Usually presents with calf claudication. Isolated femoral

Type A Endovascular treatment of choice

Type B Currently, endovascular treatment
is more often used but insufficient
evidence for recommendation

Type C Currently, surgical treatment is
more often used but insufficient
evidence for recommendation

Type D Surgical treatment of choice

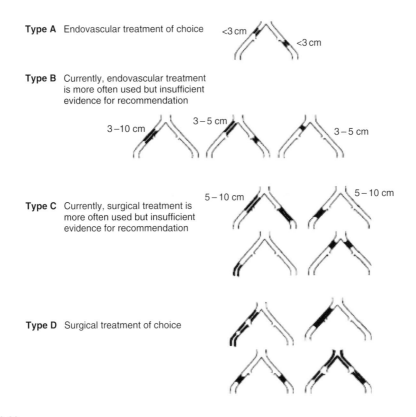

Figure 2.23

TASC classification of aorto-iliac lesions. CIA, common iliac artery; EIA, external iliac artery; CFA, common femoral artery; AAA, abdominal aortic aneurysm.

Reprinted from: Eur J Vasc Endovasc Surg, Vol. 33, Suppl. 1, Norgren L, Hiatt WR, Dormandy JA, et al. Inter-Society Consensus for the Management of Peripheral Arterial Disease (TASC II), Pages S1–S75, Copyright, 2007, with permission from Elsevier.

artery occlusion can have collateral circulation to more distal vessels and, rarely, is the cause of more advanced forms of ischemia.

  c. Runoff disease (disease in the trifurcation vessels: Anterior tibial, posterior tibial, or peroneal arteries and to the pedal arteries). These lesions are more commonly associated with limb-threatening ischemia because of the absence of collateral pathways beyond these lesions.

It is important to remember that a particular patient may have combined inflow and outflow disease.

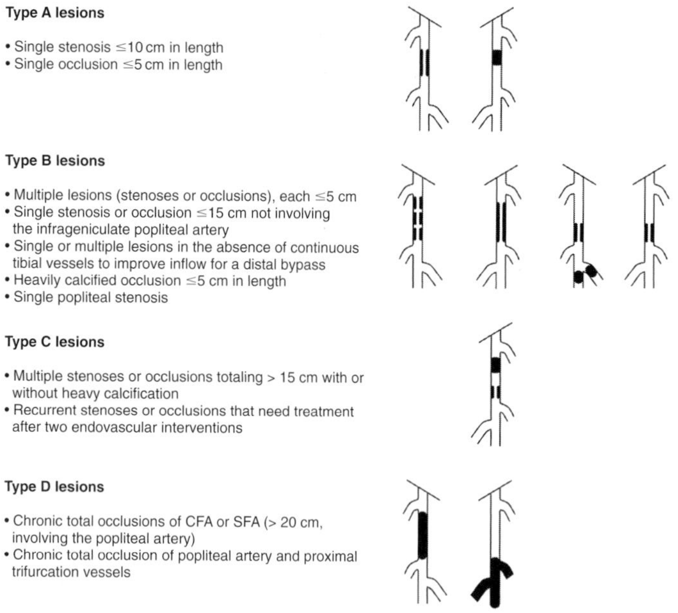

Type A lesions

- Single stenosis ≤10 cm in length
- Single occlusion ≤5 cm in length

Type B lesions

- Multiple lesions (stenoses or occlusions), each ≤5 cm
- Single stenosis or occlusion ≤15 cm not involving the infrageniculate popliteal artery
- Single or multiple lesions in the absence of continuous tibial vessels to improve inflow for a distal bypass
- Heavily calcified occlusion ≤5 cm in length
- Single popliteal stenosis

Type C lesions

- Multiple stenoses or occlusions totaling > 15 cm with or without heavy calcification
- Recurrent stenoses or occlusions that need treatment after two endovascular interventions

Type D lesions

- Chronic total occlusions of CFA or SFA (> 20 cm, involving the popliteal artery)
- Chronic total occlusion of popliteal artery and proximal trifurcation vessels

Figure 2.24

Summary of preferred options for interventional treatment of femoropopliteal lesions.

Reprinted from: J Vasc Surg, Vol. 3, Dormandy JA, Rutherford RB. Management of peripheral arterial disease. TASC working group, Pages S1–S296. Copyright, 2000, with permission from Elsevier.

Percutaneous treatment of claudication

Endovascular intervention is recommended as the preferred method of revascularization for TASC type A lesions.

In stenoses in which their hemodynamic significance is in question, it is recommended to obtain translesional pressure gradients. A gradient is considered significant if there is a peak systolic difference of 5 to 10 mmHg at baseline, or 10 to 15 mmHg after vasodilator administration.[12, 57]

Percutaneous techniques to treat PAD include percutaneous transluminal angioplasty (PTA), stent deployment, atherectomy, laser, cutting balloon angioplasty, thermal angioplasty, fibrinolysis, and thrombectomy.

Outcomes of PTA and stents depend on anatomic and clinical factors. Figure 2.26 shows different patency rates depending on the location and percutaneous approach used. Figures 2.27 and 2.28 represent patency rates and mortality comparing different surgical procedures for iliofemoral or femoropopliteal lesions. Table 2.13 summarizes several landmark randomized controlled trials of superficial femoral artery stenting.

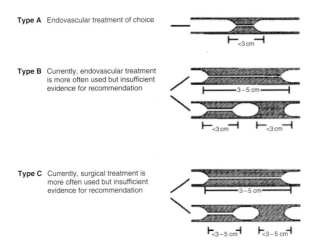

Type A Endovascular treatment of choice

Type B Currently, endovascular treatment is more often used but insufficient evidence for recommendation

Type C Currently, surgical treatment is more often used but insufficient evidence for recommendation

Figure 2.25

TASC classification of femoral popliteal lesions. CFA, common femoral artery; SFA, superficial femoral artery.

Reprinted from: Eur J Vasc Endovasc Surg, Vol. 33, Suppl. 1, Norgren L, Hiatt WR, Dormandy JA, et al. Inter-Society Consensus for the Management of Peripheral Arterial Disease (TASC II), Pages S1–S75, Copyright, 2007, with permission from Elsevier.

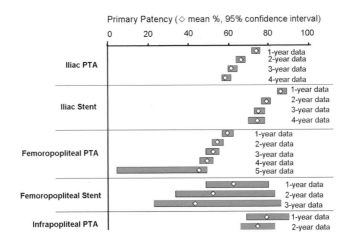

Primary Patency (◇ mean %, 95% confidence interval)

Iliac PTA	1-year data / 2-year data / 3-year data / 4-year data
Iliac Stent	1-year data / 2-year data / 3-year data / 4-year data
Femoropopliteal PTA	1-year data / 2-year data / 3-year data / 4-year data / 5-year data
Femoropopliteal Stent	1-year data / 2-year data / 3-year data
Infrapopliteal PTA	1-year data / 2-year data

Figure 2.26

Patency rates for endovascular procedures.

Adapted with information from the tables of J Vasc Interv Radiol 2001;12:683–95 (438a).

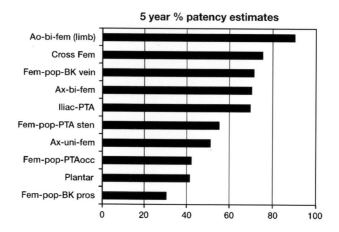

Figure 2.27

Average five-year primary patency rates for surgical revascularization. Ao-bi-fem e Aortobifemoral bypass; Cross Fem, crossover femoral graft; Fem-pop, femoropopliteal; BK, below knee; Ax-bi-fem, Axillobifemoral; PTA, Percutaneous Transluminal Angioplasty; Ax-uni-fem, Axillounifemoral bypass; pros, prosthetic.

Reprinted from: Eur J Vasc Endovasc Surg, Vol. 33, Suppl. 1, Norgren L, Hiatt WR, Dormandy JA, et al. Inter-Society Consensus for the Management of Peripheral Arterial Disease (TASC II), Pages S1–S75, Copyright, 2007, with permission from Elsevier.

Durability of patency after PTA is greatest for lesions in the common iliac artery and decreases distally. Durability also decreases with increasing length of the stenosis/occlusion, with the presence of multiple and diffuse lesions, when there is poor quality runoff, in diabetics, in patients with chronic kidney disease, in those who continue to smoke, or in patients with critical limb ischemia.

PTA can also be used to treat focal vein bypass graft stenoses, with 1- to 3-year patency rates of approximately 60% (comparable to that of surgical repair).[58] However, the 3-year patency rates of PTA for multiple vein graft stenoses are as low as 6%.[59]

A singular challenge is that of stenoses of 50%–75% angiographic diameter. Many of these lesions may not be hemodynamically significant, and intravascular pressure measurements with or without vasodilators have been recommended to determine whether these lesions are significant and to predict clinical improvement if the lesion is treated. Unfortunately, there is no consensus on diagnostic trans-stenotic pressure criteria or on methods to measure these pressures. Suggested gradients include:

- Mean gradient of 10 mmHg.[60]
- Mean gradient of 5 mmHg at rest; greater than 15 mmHg after vasodilator.[61]
- Peak systolic gradient 5 mmHg at rest; 10 to 20 mmHg after vasodilator.[12, 57]

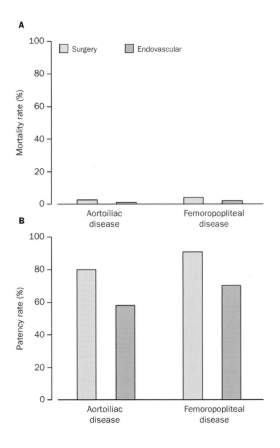

Figure 2.28

Periprocedural mortality rates and 3-year patency rates in patients undergoing percutaneous angioplasty/stenting or surgical revascularization.

Reprinted from: The Lancet, Vol. 358, Ouriel K. Peripheral arterial disease, Pages 1257–64, Copyright 2001, with permission from Elsevier.

Pressure measurements may be obtained by using two separate pressure transducers or by obtaining pull-back pressures with a single transducer. Pressures obtained with a catheter across the stenosis may artifactually increase the pressure gradient by reducing the residual lumen with the catheter. An alternative is the use of pressure wires.

Two points that merit consideration:

- Endovascular treatment of a stenosis that lacks a pressure gradient is not indicated.
- No studies have been performed to assess the safety and efficacy of treating asymptomatic but hemodynamically significant lesions to prevent progression of disease.

Table 2.13   Landmark Randomized Controlled Trials of Superficial Femoral Artery Stenting

Study, Year	N patients/ N limbs	Patient Characteristics	Inclusion Criteria and Lesion Characteristics	Exclusion Criteria	Interventions (N)	Adjunctive Therapy	Endpoints	Results
Cejna, 2001[62]	141/154	67 yo (mean) 95 limbs male 59 limbs female	Claudication, chronic limb ischemia or minor tissue loss (Categories 1–5). Up to three 5 cm SFA lesions; or proximal popliteal; at least one patent runoff vessel.	Acute thromboembolism Previous vascular surgery Untreated inflow disease	PTA (77) vs. Palmaz stent (77)	ASA 100 mg bolus and life-long thereafter. UFH 1000 U intraoperatively; continued for 24 hours	Primary: Angiography at 1 year. Secondary: procedural success; ABI: 48 hour, 3, 6 and 12 months.	Initial PTA success 84% Initial Stent success 99% 1-year angiographic patency 74% for PTA vs. 86% for stenting (P = 0.5)
Becquemin, 2003[63]	227/227	66 yo (mean) 142 male 85 female ~ 10% diabetic	Severe claudication or limb-threatening ischemia (stage IIb, III, or IV). SFA lesions 1–7 cm.	Acute ischemia Previous surgery Coagulation disorder Inflow disease	PTA (115) vs. Palmaz stent (112)	LMWH for 24 hours. Aspirin or ticlopidine lifelong	Primary: 1-year angiographic patency. Secondary: survival; vascular events.	140 angiograms available at 1-year follow-up. Restenosis in 32% for PTA and 34% for stenting (P = 0.85). No difference in survival or vascular events.
Grenacher, 2004 (REFSA trial)[64]	116/124	67 yo (mean) 78 male 38 female	Intermittent claudication or chronic limb ischemia. SFA lesions < 5 cm, at least one patent runoff vessel.	Lesions > 5 cm requiring > 2 stents Multifocal disease or total SFA occlusion Other untreated hemodynamically significant lesions Occlusion of > 2 runoff vessels Contraindications for vascular surgery or anticoagulation	PTA (53) vs. Palmaz stent (71)	ASA 100 mg bolus and UFH 5000 U intraoperatively. LMWH for 48 hours. ASA 100 mg lifelong.	Primary: long-term patency Secondary: 3, 6, 12 and 24 month follow up with angiography and duplex ultrasound; "clinical success", initial procedural success.	Initial success 94% for PTA vs. 98% for stenting. 1-year and 2-year angiographic primary patency rates were 66% and 49% in the stent group vs. 76% and 66% in the PTA group. "Clinical success" at 1 and 2 years was 80% and 77% in the PTA group versus 78.1 and 71.0% in the stent group.

Continues

Table 2.13   Landmark Randomized Controlled Trials of Superficial Femoral Artery Stenting (Continued)

STUDY, YEAR	N PATIENTS/ N LIMBS	PATIENT CHARACTERISTICS	INCLUSION CRITERIA AND LESION CHARACTERISTICS	EXCLUSION CRITERIA	INTERVENTIONS (N)	ADJUNCTIVE THERAPY	ENDPOINTS	RESULTS
Duda, 2006 (SIROCCO trial)[65]	93	66 yo (mean) 67 male 26 female ~ 40% diabetic	Symptomatic peripheral artery disease Rutherford stages 1–4, de novo or restenosis. All lesions TASC type C. Stenotic lesion length 7 to 15–20 cm (in two different phases of the study). CTO length 4 to 15–20 cm (in two different phases of the study).	Poor inflow, uremia, aneurysm of target vessel, previous stenting, ischemic tissue loss, dialysis, end-stage liver disease, recent stroke, severe vessel tortuosity or calcification, requirement of popliteal stenting, allergy to study drugs.	Nitinol stent (46) vs. Sirolimus-eluting stent (47)	ASA 300 mg pre-procedure then for 12 months. Ticlopidine or clopidogrel recommended for 4 weeks. Intraoperative UFH bolus and infusion up to 24 hours.	Primary: in-stent mean lumen diameter stenosis at 6 months as determined by quantitative angiography. Secondary: restenosis by quantitative angiography (> 50% stenosis), hemodynamic failure of the stented lesion (increase in peak systolic velocity > 100% by duplex in the stenotic segment when compared with a proximal segment or absence of a Doppler signal), ABI, clinical patency, technical and procedural success, chronic limb ischemia, serious adverse events.	No statistically significant difference in the in-stent mean lumen diameter at 6 months. 24-month restenosis rate 21.1% for nitinol vs. 22.9% for sirolimus stent (P < 0.05) Median ABI at 24 months 0.96 for sirolimus vs. 0.87 for nitinol stent (P < 0.05) Mortality, target lesion and target vessel revascularization were not significantly different in the two groups.
Schillinger, 2006 (Vienna trial)[66]	104	66 yo (mean) 55 male 49 female ~ 35% diabetic	At least Rutherford 3–5 chronic limb ischemia. SFA lesions > 3 cm, at least one patent tibioperoneal runoff vessel.	Untreated ipsilateral inflow disease Previous bypass or stent in target SFA Multiple lesions exceeding 10 cm Acute critical limb ischemia Contrast or study medication intolerance	PTA (53) vs. Nitinol stent (51)	Aspirin 100 mg daily. Clopidogrel 75 mg at least 2 days preoperatively or 300 mg loading dose intraoperatively.	Primary: rate of binary restenosis at 6 months (by computed tomography angiography or digital substraction angiography. Secondary (at 3, 6 and 12 months): Rate of restenosis by duplex; stent fractures; ABI; treadmill test; quality of life.	Restenosis rate was 43% with PTA vs. 24% with stenting (P = 0.05). Stent fracture rate 2% at one year. Walking distance significantly increased in the stent group vs. PTA group at 6 months (average distance, 363 vs. 270 m; P = 0.04) and 12 months (average distance, 387 vs. 267 m; P = 0.04). 12-month ABI better in the stent group than in the angioplasty group (~0.9 vs. ~ 0.7, P = 0.03).

Continues

Table 2.13   Landmark Randomized Controlled Trials of Superficial Femoral Artery Stenting (Continued)

Study, Year	N patients/ N limbs	Patient Characteristics	Inclusion Criteria and Lesion Characteristics	Exclusion Criteria	Interventions (N)	Adjunctive Therapy	Endpoints	Results
Kedora, 2007[67]	86/100	69 yo (mean) ~ 35% diabetic	Lifestyle-altering claudication or rest pain with or without tissue loss. SFA stenosis or occlusion, at least one vessel run-off.	Inflow disease	ePTFE or Dacron surgical graft (50) vs. ePTFE/nitinol self-expandable stent-grafting (50)	UFH 100 U/Kg intraoperatively ASA 81 to 325 mg and clopidogrel 75 mg daily at least for three months. (If patients required warfarin for other conditions, only warfarin plus ASA 81 mg)	Primary patency, secondary patency at 12 months.	No statistical difference was found in the primary patency (73% for stent-graft vs. 74% for surgery, P = 0.895) or secondary patency (P = 0.861) between the two treatment groups. Mean of 2.3 stent grafts placed per limb. Technical success 100% in both arms.
Krakenberg, 2007 (FAST Trial)[68]	244	66 yo (mean) 168 male 76 female ~ 35% diabetic ~ 35% CTO	Claudication, at least Rutherford class 2. SFA lesions 1–10 cm, at least 70% stenosis, all distal vessels patent.	Lesion requiring pretreatment (e.g., debulking) Lesion extension into popliteal artery Previous SFA stent Multiple lesions exceeding 10 cm Acute or subacute thrombotic occlusion Untreated inflow disease Ongoing dialysis or treatment with anti-platelet or anticoagulant agents	PTA (121) vs. Nitinol stent (123)	ASA 500 mg IV bolus or 100 mg 10 days prior UFH 1000–5000 U intraoperatively	Primary: Binary restenosis at 1-year, defined as proximal peak velocity ratio > 2.4 on duplex ultrasound. Secondary: 1-year target lesion revascularization, absolute walking distance, ABI, Rutherford category, major adverse events, stent integrity.	Procedural success 79% for PTA vs. 95% for stenting. 1-year primary outcome 38% for PTA vs. 31% for stenting (P = 0.3). Target lesion revascularization 18% for PTA vs. 15% for stenting. Both groups experienced similar ABI and Rutherford category improvements. Walking distance improvement was 52 m for PTA vs. 20 m for stenting (P = 0.02)

Continues

Table 2.13   Landmark Randomized Controlled Trials of Superficial Femoral Artery Stenting (Continued)

Study, Year	N patients/ N limbs	Patient Characteristics	Inclusion Criteria and Lesion Characteristics	Exclusion Criteria	Interventions (N)	Adjunctive Therapy	Endpoints	Results
Saxon, 2008[69]	197	N/A	Symptomatic peripheral arterial disease. SFA stenosis or occlusion < 13 cm in length.	N/A	PTA (100) vs. ePTFE/nitinol self expanding stent-graft (97)	N/A	Primary: 1-year patency by duplex ultrasonography. Secondary: Technical success, clinical status, major adverse events.	The stent-graft group had a significantly higher technical success rate (95% vs. 66%, P < .0001) and 1-year primary vessel patency rate (65% vs. 40%, P = .0003). A patency benefit was seen for lesions at least 3 cm long. At 12 months, chronic limb ischemia status was 15% further improved for the stent-graft group (P = .003). There were no significant differences between treatment groups with regard to the occurrence of early or late major adverse events.

Note: Most trials included only SFA lesions at least 1 cm from the origin of the SFA. All studies were unblinded randomized controlled trials, except the SIROCCO trial, which was a double blind randomized trial. Key: ABI, ankle-brachial index; ASA, Aspirin; cm, centimeters; CTO, chronic total occlusion; ePTFE, expanded polytetrafluoroethylene; IV, intravenous; LMWH, low molecular weight heparin; m, meters; N/A, not available; PTA, percutaneous transluminal angioplasty; SFA, superficial femoral artery; TASC, TransAtlantic Inter-Society Consensus; U, units; UFH, unfractionated heparin; yo, years-old.

Figures 2.29 and 2.30 show an angiogram of a patient with a TASC B iliac lesion treated with stent deployment. Figures 2.31 and 2.32 show angiograms of a TASC D femoral lesion treated with stent deployments.

Surgical treatment of claudication

Surgical revascularization is indicated for patients with claudication whose symptoms cause functional or lifestyle disruption and with unsatisfactory response to medical therapy. Two other conditions should be met for surgical revascularization to take place: Suitable arterial anatomy and a reasonable perioperative cardiovascular risk. The latter is of particular significance given the high concomitant prevalence of cardiovascular disease

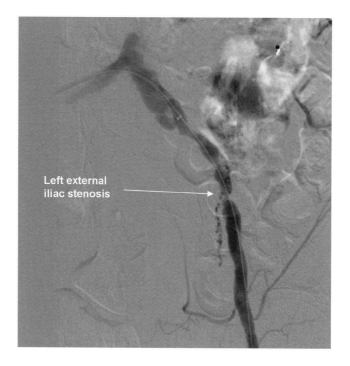

Figure 2.29

Digital substraction angiography reveals a TASC B severe iliac stenosis.

and risk factors, and because all lower extremity vascular surgical procedures have an increased risk of perioperative myocardial infarction.[11]

Perioperative Risk Assessment and Risk Reduction   A first step in pre-operative care is adequate identification of patients at risk of perioperative cardiac events. In addition to the Goldman and Detsky risk scores, the Revised Cardiac Risk Index, developed in 1999 by Lee et al., is currently the most widely used model of risk assessment in non-cardiac surgery. This index identifies six predictors of major cardiac complications: High-risk surgery, ischemic heart disease, congestive heart failure, cerebrovascular disease, insulin-dependent diabetes mellitus, and kidney disease. Based on the presence of none, one, two, or three predictors, the rate of major cardiac complications was estimated as 0.4%, 0.9%, 7%, and 11%, respectively.[70]

Once the pre-operative risk assessment indicates an increased cardiac or post-operative risk, further cardiac testing is warranted if the impact of test results would affect perioperative management. According to the 2007 guidelines of the American College of Cardiology and the American Heart Association, patients with active cardiac conditions

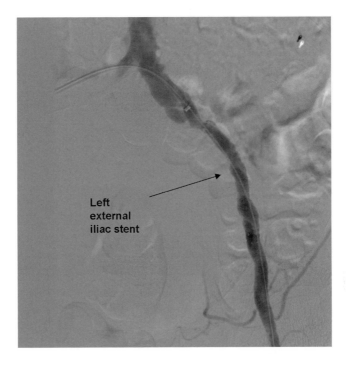

Left
external
iliac stent

Figure 2.30

Digital substraction angiography shows adequate angiographic result.

(i.e., unstable coronary syndromes, decompensated heart failure, significant arrhythmias, or severe valvular disease) should be evaluated and treated before surgery.[71]

Pre-operative cardiac testing for elective surgery is considered reasonable for patients with three clinical risk factors and poor functional capacity who require vascular surgery. It may be considered in patients with at least one to two clinical risk factors and poor functional capacity who require intermediate-risk non-cardiac surgery and in patients with at least one to two clinical risk factors and good functional capacity who are undergoing vascular surgery (Figure 2.33).[71]

Although pre-operative testing may be considered for patients with one or two risk factors scheduled for vascular surgery, the results of the randomized, multicenter DECREASE-II study suggested a different approach. If patients received beta-blockers with tight heart-rate control, the perioperative cardiac event rate was reduced. Test results and subsequent alteration in perioperative management were redundant, and there were no significant differences in cardiac death and MI at 30 days among the 770 patients studied.[72]

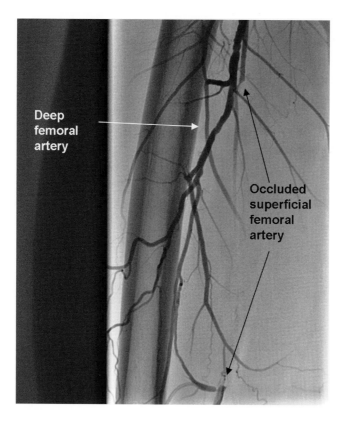

Figure 2.31

Angiography in a patient with claudication reveals an occluded right superficial femoral artery (TASC D) lesion.

Prophylactic pre-operative coronary revascularization does not appear to have a role in stable patients with PAD. The Coronary Artery Revascularization Prophylaxis (CARP) trial investigated the benefit of coronary revascularization before elective major vascular surgery, mostly in patients with one or two-vessel disease and preserved ejection fraction. In that study, 510 patients with significant coronary artery stenoses were randomized to either revascularization or no revascularization before vascular surgery. There was no reduction in the number of myocardial infarctions, deaths, hospital stay, or long-term outcomes.[73]

In a recent study evaluating vascular surgery patients with predominantly three-vessel coronary disease, similar findings were obtained: The incidence of a composite endpoint of all-cause mortality and MI at 30 days was 43% in the revascularized coronary group versus 33% (OR 1.4, 95% CI 0.7 to 2.8, p = 0.30).[74]

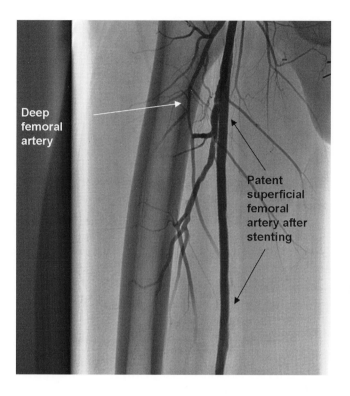

Figure 2.32

Angiography after successful stenting with two overlapping covered stents.

Type of Surgery	Functional Capacity	Number of Clinical Risk Factors
		0 1 2 3 ≥4
Vascular Surgery	Good	
	Poor	
Intermediate Risk Surgery	Good	
	Poor	
Low Risk Surgery	Good	
	Poor	

Figure 2.33

Recommendations for Noninvasive Stress Testing According to the ACC/AHA Guidelines (2007): Light gray bars indicate no recommendation of noninvasive stress testing and that patients can go directly to surgery; dark gray bars indicate patients for whom testing may be considered if it will change management (class IIb); and the white bar indicates a class IIa recommendation for noninvasive stress testing. ACC/AHA = American College of Cardiology/American Heart Association.

Reprinted from: J Am Coll Cardiol, Vol. 51, Poldermans D, Hoeks SE, Feringa HH. Pre-operative risk assessment and risk reduction before surgery, Pages 1813–24, Copyright, 2008, with permission from Elsevier.

The optimal pre-operative management of patients with left main disease, severe left ventricular dysfunction, unstable angina, and aortic stenosis has not been determined. However, both of the studies described above suggest that prophylactic coronary revascularization of cardiac-stable patients provides no benefit for immediate post-operative outcome. In accordance with this evidence, the new ACC/AHA guidelines indicate that routine prophylactic coronary revascularization is not recommended in patients with *stable* CAD before non-cardiac surgery.[71]

Another important clinical situation is the management of patients with previous coronary stenting undergoing non-cardiac surgery. The risk of perioperative stent thrombosis in these patients is increased by the non-cardiac surgical procedure, especially when surgery is performed early after stent implantation and particularly if dual antiplatelet therapy is discontinued. When possible, it is advised to delay surgery until after the time window that requires dual antiplatelet therapy. The new ACC/AHA guidelines recommend, based on expert opinion, 30–45 days for bare-metal stents and 1 year for drug-eluting stents.[71]

In most patients, perioperative use of beta-blockers is associated with reduced cardiovascular risk of surgery. Recent studies have shown that treatment with bisoprolol significantly decreased the risk for cardiovascular events during vascular surgery and afterwards. Besides controlling symptoms of myocardial ischemia, treatment with beta-blocking agents also has the benefit of favorably influencing prognosis in these patients (Figure 2.34). A recent large meta-analysis by Schouten et al. included 15 studies (1,077 patients) and showed a significant beneficial effect of beta-blockers in non-cardiac surgery patients.[75–79]

Different large clinical trials in patients with CAD have shown a beneficial effect of statins (Figure 2.35). The 4S trial demonstrated that simvastatin improved outcomes

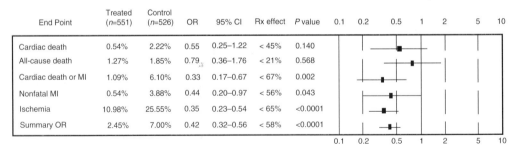

End Point	Treated (*n*=551)	Control (*n*=526)	OR	95% CI	Rx effect	*P* value
Cardiac death	0.54%	2.22%	0.55	0.25–1.22	< 45%	0.140
All-cause death	1.27%	1.85%	0.79	0.36–1.76	< 21%	0.568
Cardiac death or MI	1.09%	6.10%	0.33	0.17–0.67	< 67%	0.002
Nonfatal MI	0.54%	3.88%	0.44	0.20–0.97	< 56%	0.043
Ischemia	10.98%	25.55%	0.35	0.23–0.54	< 65%	<0.0001
Summary OR	2.45%	7.00%	0.42	0.32–0.56	< 58%	<0.0001

Figure 2.34

Pooled effect of perioperative beta-blockers.

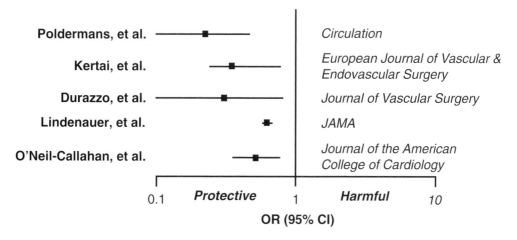

Figure 2.35

Effects in cardiovascular outcomes with perioperative statin use.

Reprinted from: J Am Coll Cardiol, Vol. 51, Poldermans D, Hoeks SE, Feringa HH. Pre-operative risk assessment and risk reduction before surgery, Pages 1813–24, Copyright, 2008, with permission from Elsevier.

in patients with CAD. It also showed that simvastatin use was also associated with a reduction of new or worsening intermittent claudication. These observations are consistent in patients undergoing vascular surgery.[79]

Aspirin is one of the cornerstones in the primary and secondary prevention of cardiovascular diseases. The evidence of ASA in the perioperative period in patients undergoing non-cardiac surgery is not very clear. A meta-analysis demonstrated a reduction of serious vascular events and vascular death in patients with peripheral vascular disease. That study included 10 trials of antiplatelet treatment in lower limb bypass surgery, of which six involved ASA treatment. However, the benefit of antiplatelet therapy did not reach statistical significance for the combined endpoint of vascular events (OR 0.76, 95% CI 0.54 to 1.05) in that vascular surgery population.[80]

Concerns of promoting perioperative hemorrhagic complications often lead to ASA withholding in the perioperative period. There are no randomized controlled trials on pre-operative discontinuation of ASA. A systematic review in subjects at risk for or with known CAD demonstrated that ASA non-adherence or withdrawal was associated with a three-fold higher risk of major adverse cardiac events (OR 3.14, 95% CI 1.75 to 5.61; p = 0.0001).[81]

Inflow procedures   As described above, surgical procedures are subdivided into inflow, outflow, or runoff disease revascularizations.

Table 2.14 provides certain characteristics of different inflow procedures, and Figures 2.36 and 2.37 show an angiogram of a patient who may likely benefit from an

Table 2.14   Vascular Surgical Procedures for Inflow Improvement

Inflow Procedure	Operative Mortality (%)	Expected Patency Rate (%)
Aortobifemoral bypass	3.3	87.5 (5 years)
Aortoiliac or aortofemoral bypass	1–2	85–90 (5 years)
Iliac endarterectomy	0	79–90 (5 years)
Femorofemoral bypass	6	71 (5 years)
Axillofemoral bypass	6	49–80 (3 years)
Axillofemoral-femoral bypass	4.9	63–67.7 (5 years)

Table adapted with information obtained from reference 11.

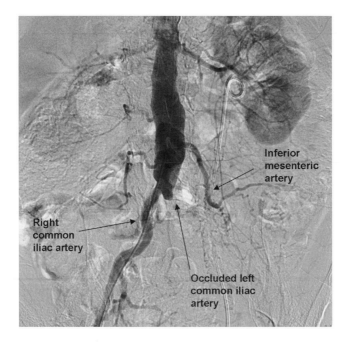

Figure 2.36

Digital substraction angiography in a patient with severe aortoiliac disease who may benefit from an inflow procedure.

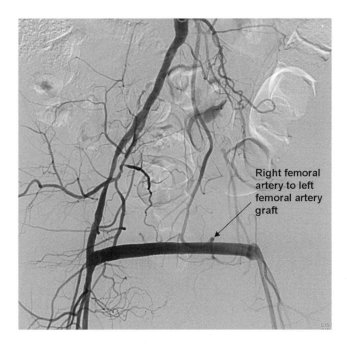

Right femoral artery to left femoral artery graft

Figure 2.37

Digital substraction angiography in a patient with severe left-sided aortoiliac disease and a right femoral to left femoral graft.

inflow procedure, and an angiogram of a patient post-procedure. Inflow procedures are performed using artificial grafts (polyester or polytetrafluoroethylene).

Aortobifemoral bypass is performed through a transabdominal or a retroperitoneal approach, and is constructed by suturing (typically end-to-end) the proximal end of a bifurcated graft to the aorta, immediately below the origin of the renal arteries. The distal graft limbs are sutured to the distal common femoral arteries or onto the proximal deep femoral arteries (Figure 2.38).

Patients with severe infrarenal aortic atherosclerosis who are at high cardiovascular or surgical risk for open aortobifemoral bypass may be treated with axillofemoral-femoral bypass (Figure 2.39).

Outflow procedures   Outflow procedures can be performed under general or regional anesthesia and are better tolerated than inflow procedures.

Most studies have shown that patency rates are increased if vein conduits are used. This is true for both above-the-knee and below-the-knee grafts. Therefore, artificial grafts are only used if veins are absent or inadequate for grafting.

Table 2.15 provides more details on outflow procedures and their outcomes. Figures 2.40 and 2.41 depict common outflow grafts.

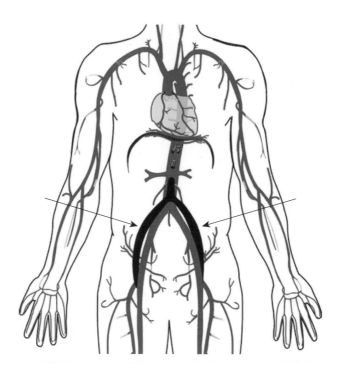

Figure 2.38

Bilateral bypass from infra renal abdominal aorta to both femoral arteries (arrows indicate bypass graft).

Reprinted from: Eur J Vasc Endovasc Surg, Vol. 33, Suppl. 1, Norgren L, Hiatt WR, Dormandy JA, et al. Inter-Society Consensus for the Management of Peripheral Arterial Disease (TASC II), Pages S1–S75, Copyright, 2007, with permission from Elsevier.

Treatment of Critical and Acute Limb Ischemia

Acute limb ischemia is a medical emergency, as restoration of blood flow may save the limb. Critical limb ischemia, on the other hand, is usually due to progression of chronic PAD, but restoration of flow can also lead to limb salvage.

Patients with acute or critical limb ischemia should undergo immediate angiography to provide adequate delineation of the anatomy jeopardizing limb viability or to perform supraselective intra-arterial thrombolysis. Table 2.16 provides clues to the stratification of limb threat by viability; Figures 2.42 and 2.43 provide general algorithms that may be used in the evaluation of these patients.

Selective or supraselective thrombolysis guided by catheter (more effective and with decreased complications when compared to systemic thrombolysis), as well as adjunctive mechanical thrombectomy, are indicated in patients with acute limb ischemia Rutherford

If these interventions are not feasible or fail, it may be necessary to amputate the extremity. Table 2.19 summarizes indications for amputation after failed thrombolysis or surgery.

Amputation is not a benign surgical procedure. It is associated with a 30-day mortality risk of 4%–30% and a 20%–40% risk of morbidity, including myocardial infarction, stroke, and infection.[11, 12]

Follow-Up Surveillance After Intervention

In order to maximize the benefit of revascularization and to minimize the overall cardiovascular risk, all postoperative patients with PAD should be maintained on maximal cardiovascular ischemic risk reduction therapies whenever possible (ACE inhibitors, statins, beta-blockers) and should be maintained on antiplatelet agents. These patients should be considered in the highest cardiovascular risk category and warrant aggressive risk factor modification.

A follow-up surveillance program is imperative for patients undergoing both percutaneous and surgical revascularization. Table 2.20 provides recommended follow-up guidelines. There is no evidence regarding the most adequate follow-up intervals, but consideration should be given to the initial clinical presentation, the burden of disease, and the type of procedure (aortic and common iliac artery procedures have greater durability than infrainguinal procedures, therefore requiring less frequent surveillance).

The recommendations are surveillance immediately postoperatively and every 6 months for 2 years. Surveillance evaluation should include:[11, 12]

- Interval history and new symptoms
- Vascular examination of the leg with palpation of proximal, graft, and outflow vessel pulses
- Periodic measurement of resting and, if possible, postexercise ankle-brachial indices

Table 2.19   Indications for Amputation

Necrosis of the weight-bearing portions of the foot (if patient is ambulatory)
Uncorrectable flexion contracture
Paresis of the extremity
Refractory ischemic rest pain
Sepsis
Very limited life expectancy due to comorbid conditions

Table 2.20   Surveillance Programs for Different Revascularization Procedures

Patients undergoing revascularization of the lower extremity should be entered into a surveillance program that consists of:

- Interval history (new symptoms)
- Vascular examination of the leg with palpation of proximal and outflow vessel pulses (and graft pulses if grafted)
- Resting and, if possible, postexercise ABI recording

Aortoiliac and infrainguinal transluminal angioplasty

Surveillance should be performed in the immediate post-PTA period and at intervals for at least 2 years

Infrainguinal prosthetic grafts

Surveillance should be performed in the immediate postoperative period and at regular intervals (timing of surveillance and efficacy have not been ideally defined) for at least 2 years

Infrainguinal vein bypass grafts

- Also, duplex scanning of the entire length of the graft, with calculation of peak systolic velocities and velocity ratios across all identified lesions
- Surveillance programs should be performed in the immediate postoperative period and at regular intervals for at least 2 years
- Femoral-popliteal and femoral-tibial venous conduit bypass at approximately 3, 6, and 12 months and annually thereafter

Adapted with information from reference 11.

Although recommended by the ACC and TASC I guidelines, the newest TASC II guidelines do not formally recommend vein graft surveillance with duplex scanning (still present in Table 2.20).[11, 12] The purpose was to identify lesions that predisposed patients to graft thrombosis and allow repair prior to graft occlusion. However, a recent multicenter randomized controlled trial showed that duplex surveillance after venous femoral distal bypass grafts leads to no significant clinical benefit.[91] Many centers, however, continue with vein graft surveillance programs while awaiting confirmation of the findings of this trial. Because duplex imaging is of limited benefit for the detection of lesions within synthetic grafts, recording of ABIs has been considered sufficient in patients with synthetic grafts.

If patients have an abnormal physical exam or ABIs, Doppler evaluation is recommended. Prompt evaluation with angiography is then indicated when non-invasive methods suggest hemodynamically significant lesions (> 50% stenosis).

In the case of percutaneous procedures, the role of surveillance is less well established. Regular visits, with assessment of interval change in symptoms, vascular examination, and ABI measurement, are considered the standard of care. Postexercise ABI determinations may be useful in some individuals. The utility and role of duplex ultrasound and other non-invasive diagnostic modalities (MRA and CTA) for such routine surveillance of endovascular sites have yet to be determined.

There is no uniformly accepted threshold for repeat angiography and intervention in the patient with evidence of recurrent stenosis. Patients who have recurrent symptoms in association with evidence of hemodynamic compromise require restudy and repeat intervention. Likewise, evidence of rapidly progressive restenosis, even in the absence of symptoms, should provide a clue that may identify individuals who might benefit from future invasive management.

For grafts, as well as native vessels, a stenosis of less than 50% appears to be associated with favorable prognosis and patency. In contrast, a stenosis greater than 70% is a harbinger of poor long-term patency, and thus, reintervention may be warranted.[11]

Cost effectiveness

A cost-effectiveness analysis compared PTA and bypass surgery with exercise therapy for the treatment of claudication. The cost effectiveness of PTA was $38,000 for quality-adjusted life year (in the range of other accepted procedures). Bypass surgery cost-effectiveness was $311,000 per quality-adjusted life year.[92]

REFERENCES

1. Criqui MH, Fronek A, Barrett-Connor E, Klauber MR, Gabriel S, Goodman D. The prevalence of peripheral arterial disease in a defined population. *Circulation.* 1985;71:510–515.

2. Diehm C, Schuster A, Allenberg JR, et al. High prevalence of peripheral arterial disease and co-morbidity in 6880 primary care patients: cross-sectional study. *Atherosclerosis.* 2004;172:95–105.

3. Hirsch AT, Criqui MH, Treat-Jacobson D, et al. Peripheral arterial disease detection, awareness, and treatment in primary care. *JAMA.* 2001;286:1317–1324.

4. Selvin E, Erlinger TP. Prevalence of and risk factors for peripheral arterial disease in the United States: results from the National Health and Nutrition Examination Survey, 1999–2000. *Circulation.* 2004; 110:738–743.

5. Murabito JM, D'Agostino RB, Silbershatz H, Wilson WF. Intermittent claudication: a risk profile from The Framingham Heart Study. *Circulation.* 1997;96:44–49.

6. Newman AB, Sutton-Tyrrell K, Vogt MT, Kuller LH. Morbidity and mortality in hypertensive adults with a low ankle/arm blood pressure index. *JAMA.* 1993; 270:487–489.

7. Meijer WT, Hoes AW, Rutgers D, Bots ML, Hofman A, Grobbee DE. Peripheral arterial disease in the elderly: the Rotterdam Study. *Arterioscler Thromb Vasc Biol.* 1998;18:185–192.

8. Smith GD, Shipley MJ, Rose G. Intermittent claudication, heart disease risk factors, and mortality: the Whitehall Study. *Circulation.* 1990;82:1925–1931.

9. Fowkes FG, Housley E, Cawood EH, Macintyre CC, Ruckley CV, Prescott RJ. Edinburgh Artery Study: prevalence of asymptomatic and symptomatic peripheral arterial disease in the general population. *Int J Epidemiol.* 1991;20:384–392.

10. O'Hare AM, Vittinghoff E, Hsia J, Shlipak MG. Renal insufficiency and the risk of lower extremity peripheral arterial disease: results from the Heart and Estrogen/Progestin Replacement Study (HERS). *J Am Soc Nephrol.* 2004;15:1046–1051.

11. Hirsch AT, Haskal ZJ, Hertzer NR, et al. ACC/ AHA 2005 practice guidelines for the management of patients with peripheral arterial disease (lower extremity, renal, mesenteric, and abdominal aortic): a collaborative report from the American Association for Vascular Surgery/Society for Vascular Surgery, Society for Cardiovascular Angiography and Interventions, Society for Vascular Medicine and Biology, Society of Interventional Radiology, and the ACC/AHA Task Force on Practice Guidelines (Writing Committee to Develop Guidelines for the Management of Patients with Peripheral Arterial Disease): Endorsed by the American Association of Cardiovascular and Pulmonary Rehabilitation; National Heart, Lung, and Blood Institute; Society for Vascular Nursing; TransAtlan-

tic Inter-Society Consensus; and Vascular Disease Foundation. *Circulation.* 2006;113:e463–e654.

12. Norgren L, Hiatt WR, Dormandy JA, et al. Inter-society consensus for the management of peripheral arterial disease (TASC II). *Eur J Vasc Endovasc Surg.* 2007;33(Suppl 1):S1–S75.

13. White C. Clinical practice: intermittent claudication. *N Engl J Med.* 2007;356:1241–1250.

14. Dormandy JA, Rutherford RB. Management of peripheral arterial disease (PAD). TASC Working Group. TransAtlantic Inter-Society Consensus (TASC). *J Vasc Surg.* 2000;31:S1–S296.

15. Khan NA, Rahim SA, Anand SS, Simel DL, Panju A. Does the clinical examination predict lower extremity peripheral arterial disease? *JAMA.* 2006;295:536–546.

16. Symes JF, Graham AM, Mousseau M. Doppler waveform analysis versus segmental pressure and pulse-volume recording: assessment of occlusive disease in the lower extremity. *Can J Surg.* 1984;27: 345–347.

17. McPhail IR, Spittell PC, Weston SA, Bailey KR. Intermittent claudication: an objective office-based assessment. *J Am Coll Cardiol.* 2001;37:1381–1385.

18. Mattos MA, van Bemmelen PS, Hodgson KJ, Ramsey DE, Barkmeier LD, Sumner DS. Does correction of stenoses identified with color duplex scanning improve infrainguinal graft patency? *J Vasc Surg.* 1993;17:54–64.

19. Willmann JK, Mayer D, Banyai M, et al. Evaluation of peripheral arterial bypass grafts with multidetector row CT angiography: comparison with duplex US and digital subtraction angiography. *Radiology.* 2003;229:465–474.

20. Nelemans PJ, Leiner T, de Vet HC, van Engelshoven JM. Peripheral arterial disease: meta-analysis of the diagnostic performance of MR angiography. *Radiology.* 2000;217:105–114.

21. Loewe C, Cejna M, Schoder M, et al. Contrast material-enhanced, moving-table MR angiography versus digital subtraction angiography for surveillance of peripheral arterial bypass grafts. *J Vasc Interv Radiol.* 2003;14:1129–1137.

22. Muluk SC, Muluk VS, Kelley ME, et al. Outcome events in patients with claudication: a 15-year study in 2777 patients. *J Vasc Surg.* 2001;33:251–257.

23. Aquino R, Johnnides C, Makaroun M, et al. Natural history of claudication: long-term serial follow-up study of 1244 claudicants. *J Vasc Surg.* 2001;34: 962–970.

24. Nickenig G, Böhm M, Miche E, et al. Physical training increases endothelial progenitor cells, inhibits neointima formation, and enhances angiogenesis. *Circulation.* 2004;109:220.

25. Hirsch A, Regensteiner J, Hiatt W, Stewart K. Exercise training for claudication. *N Engl J Med.* 2002;347:1941.

26. Bendermacher BL, Willigendael EM, Teijink JA, Prins MH. Supervised exercise therapy versus nonsupervised exercise therapy for intermittent claudication. *Cochrane Database Syst Rev.* 2006;(2):CD005263.

27. Leng GC, Fowler B, Ernst E. Exercise for intermittent claudication. *Cochrane Database Syst Rev.* 2000;(2):CD000990.

28. McDermott MM, Ades P, Guralnik JM, et al. Treadmill exercise and resistance training in patients with peripheral arterial disease with and without intermittent claudication: a randomized controlled trial. *JAMA.* 2009;301:165–174.

29. Robless P, Mikhailidis DP, Stansby GP. Cilostazol for peripheral arterial disease. *Cochrane Database Syst Rev.* 2008;(1):CD003748.

30. Antithrombotic Trialists' Collaboration. Collaborative meta-analysis of randomised trials of antiplatelet therapy for prevention of death, myocardial infarction, and stroke in high risk patients. *BMJ.* 2002; 324:71–86.

31. Collaborative overview of randomised trials of antiplatelet therapy—I: Prevention of death, myocardial infarction, and stroke by prolonged antiplatelet therapy in various categories of patients. Antiplatelet Trialists' Collaboration. *BMJ.* 1994;308:81–106.

32. Girolami B, Bernardi E, Prins MH, et al. Antithrombotic drugs in the primary medical management of intermittent claudication: a meta-analysis. *Thromb Haemost.* 1999;81:715–722.

33. Bhatt DL, Fox KA, Hacke W, et al. Clopidogrel and aspirin versus aspirin alone for the prevention of atherothrombotic events. *N Engl J Med.* 2006;354: 1706–1717.

34. Dutch Bypass Oral anticoagulants or Aspirin (BOA) Study Group. Efficacy of oral anticoagulants compared with aspirin after infrainguinal bypass surgery (The Dutch Bypass Oral Anticoagulants or Aspirin Study): a randomised trial. *Lancet.* 2000;355:346–351.

35. Warfarin Antiplatelet Vascular Evaluation Trial Investigators, Anand S, Yusuf S, et al. Oral anticoagulant and antiplatelet therapy and peripheral arterial disease. *N Engl J Med.* 2007;357:217–227.

36. Anand SS, Yusuf S. Oral anticoagulants in patients with coronary artery disease. *J Am Coll Cardiol.* 2003;41:62S–69S.

37. Joint National Committee on Prevention, Detection, Evaluation and Treatment of High Blood Pressure. JNC VII. *JAMA.* 2003;289:2560–2572.

38. Radack K, Deck C. Beta-adrenergic blocker therapy does not worsen intermittent claudication in subjects

with peripheral arterial disease: a meta-analysis of randomized controlled trials. *Arch Intern Med.* 1991;151:1769–1776.

39. Yusuf S, Sleight P, Pogue J, et al. Effects of angiotensin-converting enzyme inhibitor, ramipril, on cardiovascular events in high-risk patients. *N Engl J Med.* 2000;342:145–153.

40. Heart Protection Study Collaborative Group. MRC/BHF Heart Protection Study of cholesterol lowering with simvastatin in 20,536 high-risk individuals: a randomised placebo-controlled trial. *Lancet.* 2002;360:7–22.

41. Executive Summary of the Third Report of the National Cholesterol Education Program (NCEP) Expert Panel on Detection, Evaluation, and Treatment of High Blood Cholesterol in Adults (Adult Treatment Panel III). *JAMA.* 2001;285:2486–2497.

42. Mohler ER, 3rd, Hiatt WR, Creager MA. Cholesterol reduction with atorvastatin improves walking distance in patients with peripheral arterial disease. *Circulation.* 2003;108:1481–1486.

43. Mondillo S, Ballo P, Barbati R, et al. Effects of simvastatin on walking performance and symptoms of intermittent claudication in hypercholesterolemic patients with peripheral vascular disease. *Am J Med.* 2003;114:359–364.

44. Blankenhorn DH, Azen SP, Crawford DW, et al. Effects of colestipol-niacin therapy on human femoral atherosclerosis. *Circulation.* 1991;83:438–447.

45. Wittlinger T, Kroger K. Role of lipid lowering therapy in patients with peripheral arterial occlusive disease. *Herz.* 2004;29:12–16.

46. Sprecher DL. Raising high-density lipoprotein cholesterol with niacin and fibrates: a comparative review. *Am J Cardiol.* 2000;86:46L–50L.

47. The Diabetes Control and Complications Trial (DCCT) Research Group. Effect of intensive diabetes management on macrovascular events and risk factors in the Diabetes Control and Complications Trial. *Am J Cardiol.* 1995;75:894.

48. UK Prospective Diabetes Study (UKPDS) Group. Intensive blood-glucose control with sulphonylureas or insulin compared with conventional treatment and risk of complications in patients with type 2 diabetes (UKPDS 33). *Lancet.* 1998;352:837.

49. Taton J, Smith U, Skrha J, et al. Secondary prevention of macrovascular events in patients with type 2 diabetes in the PROactive Study (PROspective pioglitAzone Clinical Trial In macroVascular Events): a randomised controlled trial. *Lancet.* 2005;366:1279.

50. De Backer TL, Vander Stichele R, Lehert P, Van Bortel L. Naftidrofuryl for intermittent claudication. *Cochrane Database Syst Rev.* 2008;(2):CD001368.

51. Brevetti G, Diehm C, Lambert D. European multicenter study on propionyl-L-carnitine in intermittent claudication. *J Am Coll Cardiol.* 1999;34:1618–1624.

52. Hiatt WR, Regensteiner JG, Creager MA, et al. Propionyl-L-carnitine improves exercise performance and functional status in patients with claudication. *Am J Med.* 2001;110:616–622.

53. Girolami B, Bernardi E, Prins MH, et al. Treatment of intermittent claudication with physical training, smoking cessation, pentoxifylline, or nafronyl: a meta-analysis. *Arch Intern Med.* 1999;159:337–345.

54. Coffman JD. Drug therapy: vasodilator drugs in peripheral vascular disease. *N Engl J Med.* 1979; 300:713–717.

55. Lederman RJ, Mendelsohn FO, Anderson RD, et al. Therapeutic angiogenesis with recombinant fibroblast growth factor-2 for intermittent claudication (the TRAFFIC study): a randomised trial. *Lancet.* 2002;359:2053–2058.

56. Isner JM, Rivard A. Angiogenesis and vasculogenesis in treatment of cardiovascular disease. *Mol Med.* 1998;4:429.

57. Rose SC, Kinney TB. Intraarterial pressure measurements during angiographic evaluation of peripheral vascular disease: techniques, interpretation, applications, and limitations. *AJR Am J Roentgenol.* 1996;166:277.

58. Avino AJ, Bandyk DF, Gonsalves AJ, et al. Surgical and endovascular intervention for infrainguinal vein graft stenosis. *J Vasc Surg.* 1999;29:60–70.

59. Whittemore AD, Donaldson MC, Polak JF, Mannick JA. Limitations of balloon angioplasty for vein graft stenosis. *J Vasc Surg.* 1991;14:340–345.

60. Mali WP, van der Graaf Y, Tielbeek AV, Spithoven JH, van Engelen AD, Tetteroo E. Stent placement after iliac angioplasty: comparison of hemodynamic and angiographic criteria. Dutch Iliac Stent Trial Study Group. *Radiology.* 1996;201:155.

61. Darling RC, O'Hara PJ, Waltman AC, Brewster DC. Femoral artery pressure measurement during aortography. *Circulation.* 1979;60:120.

62. Cejna M, Thurnher S, Illiasch H, Horvath W, Waldenberger P, Hornik K, et al. PTA versus Palmaz stent placement in femoropopliteal artery obstructions: a multicenter prospective randomized study. *J Vasc Interv Radiol.* 2001;12:23–31. [Abstract]

63. Becquemin JP, Favre JP, Marzelle J, Nemoz C, Corsin C, Leizorovicz A. Systematic versus selective stent placement after superficial femoral artery balloon angioplasty: a multicenter prospective randomized study. *J Vasc Surg.* 2003;37:487–494.

64. Grenacher L, Saam T, Geier A, Muller-Hulsbeck S, Cejna M, Kauffmann GW, et al. PTA versus Palmaz stent placement in femoropopliteal artery stenoses: results of a multicenter prospective randomized study (REFSA) [PTA versus Stent bei Stenosen der A. femoralis und A. poplitea: Ergebnisse einer prospektiv randomisierten Multizenterstudie (REFSA)]. *Fortschr Geb Rontgenstr*. 2004;176:1302–1310. [Abstract]

65. Duda SH, Bosiers M, Lammer J, et al. Drug-eluting and bare nitinol stents for the treatment of atherosclerotic lesions in the superficial femoral artery: long-term results from the SIROCCO Trial. *J Vasc Interv Radiol*. 2005 Mar;16(3):331–8. [Abstract]

66. Schillinger M, Sabeti S, Loewe C, Dick P, Amighi J, Mlekusch W, et al. Balloon angioplasty versus implantation of nitinol stents in the superficial femoral artery. *New Engl J Med*. 2006;354:1879–1888.

67. Kedora J, Hohmann S, Garrett W, Munschaur C, Theune B, Gable D. Randomized comparison of percutaneous Viabahn stent grafts vs. prosthetic femoral-popliteal bypass in the treatment of superficial femoral arterial occlusive disease. *J Vasc Surg*. 2007;45:10–16.

68. Krankenberg H, Schluter M, Steinkamp HJ, Burgelin K, Scheinert D, Schulte KL, et al. Nitinol stent implantation versus percutaneous transluminal angioplasty in superficial femoral artery lesions up to 10 cm in length: the femoral artery stenting trial (FAST). *Circulation*. 2007;116:285–292.

69. Saxon RR, Dake MD, Volgelzang RL, Katzen BT, Becker GJ. Randomized, multicenter study comparing expanded polytetrafluoroethylene-covered endoprosthesis placement with percutaneous transluminal angioplasty in the treatment of superficial femoral artery occlusive disease. *J Endovasc Ther*. 2006;13:701–710. [Abstract]

70. Lee TH, Marcantonio ER, Mangione CM, et al. Derivation and prospective validation of a simple index for prediction of cardiac risk of major noncardiac surgery. *Circulation*. 1999;100:1043–1049.

71. Fleisher LA, Beckman JA, Brown KA, et al. ACC/AHA 2007 guidelines on perioperative cardiovascular evaluation and care for noncardiac surgery: A report of the American College of Cardiology/American Heart Association Task Force on Practice Guidelines (Writing Committee to Revise the 2002 Guidelines on Perioperative Cardiovascular Evaluation for Noncardiac Surgery) developed in collaboration with the American Society of Echocardiography, American Society of Nuclear Cardiology, Heart Rhythm Society, Society of Cardiovascular Anesthesiologists, Society for Cardiovascular Angiography and Interventions, Society for Vascular Medicine and Biology, and Society for Vascular Surgery. *J Am Coll Cardiol*. 2007;50:e159–e241.

72. Poldermans D, Bax JJ, Schouten O, et al. Should major vascular surgery be delayed because of preoperative cardiac testing in intermediate-risk patients receiving beta-blocker therapy with tight heart rate control? *J Am Coll Cardiol*. 2006;48:964–969.

73. McFalls EO, Ward HB, Moritz TE, et al. Coronary-artery revascularization before elective major vascular surgery. *N Engl J Med*. 2004;351:2795–2804.

74. Poldermans D, Schouten O, Vidakovic R, et al. A clinical randomized trial to evaluate the safety of a non-invasive approach in high-risk patients undergoing major vascular surgery: The DECREASE-V Pilot Study. *J Am Coll Cardiol*. 2007;49:1763–1769.

75. Poldermans D, Boersma E, Bax JJ, et al. Bisoprolol reduces cardiac death and myocardial infarction in high-risk patients as long as 2 years after successful major vascular surgery. *Eur Heart J*. 2001;22:1353–1358.

76. Poldermans D, Boersma E, Bax JJ, et al. The effect of bisoprolol on perioperative mortality and myocardial infarction in high-risk patients undergoing vascular surgery. Dutch Echocardiographic Cardiac Risk Evaluation Applying Stress Echocardiography Study Group. *N Engl J Med*. 1999;341:1789–1794.

77. Kertai MD, Boersma E, Bax JJ, et al. Optimizing long-term cardiac management after major vascular surgery: Role of beta-blocker therapy, clinical characteristics, and dobutamine stress echocardiography to optimize long-term cardiac management after major vascular surgery. *Arch Intern Med*. 2003;163:2230–2235.

78. Schouten O, Shaw LJ, Boersma E, et al. A meta-analysis of safety and effectiveness of perioperative beta-blocker use for the prevention of cardiac events in different types of noncardiac surgery. *Coron Artery Dis*. 2006;17:173–179.

79. Pedersen TR, Kjekshus J, Pyorala K, et al. Effect of simvastatin on ischemic signs and symptoms in the Scandinavian simvastatin survival study (4S). *Am J Cardiol*. 1998;81:333–335.

80. Robless P, Mikhailidis DP, Stansby G. Systematic review of antiplatelet therapy for the prevention of myocardial infarction, stroke or vascular death in patients with peripheral vascular disease. *Br J Surg*. 2001;88:787–800.

81. Biondi-Zoccai GG, Lotrionte M, Agostoni P, et al. A systematic review and meta-analysis on the hazards of discontinuing or not adhering to aspirin among 50, 279 patients at risk for coronary artery disease. *Eur Heart J*. 2006;27:2667–2674.

82. Diffin DC, Kandarpa K. Assessment of peripheral intraarterial thrombolysis versus surgical revascularization in acute lower-limb ischemia: a review of limb-salvage and mortality statistics. *J Vasc Interv Radiol.* 1996;7:57–63.

83. Ouriel K, Shortell CK, DeWeese JA, et al. A comparison of thrombolytic therapy with operative revascularization in the initial treatment of acute peripheral arterial ischemia. *J Vasc Surg.* 1994;19:1021–1030.

84. The STILE Investigators. Results of a prospective randomized trial evaluating surgery versus thrombolysis for ischemia of the lower extremity. The STILE trial. *Ann Surg.* 1994;220:251–266.

85. Ouriel K, Veith FJ, Sasahara AA. A comparison of recombinant urokinase with vascular surgery as initial treatment for acute arterial occlusion of the legs. Thrombolysis or Peripheral Arterial Surgery (TOPAS) Investigators. *N Engl J Med.* 1998;338:1105–1111.

86. Mahler F, Schneider E, Hess H, Steering Committe, Study on Local Thrombolysis. Recombinant tissue plasminogen activator versus urokinase for local thrombolysis of femoropopliteal occlusions: a prospective, randomized multicenter trial. *J Endovasc Ther.* 2001;8:638–647.

87. Drescher P, McGuckin J, Rilling WS, Crain MR. Catheter-directed thrombolytic therapy in peri-pheral artery occlusions: combining reteplase and abciximab. *AJR Am J Roentgenol.* 2003;180:1385–1391.

88. Burkart DJ, Borsa JJ, Anthony JP, Thurlo SR. Thrombolysis of acute peripheral arterial and venous occlusions with tenecteplase and eptifibatide: a pilot study. *J Vasc Interv Radiol.* 2003;14:729–733.

89. Duda SH, Tepe G, Luz O, et al. Peripheral artery occlusion: Treatment with abciximab plus urokinase versus with urokinase alone—a randomized pilot trial (the PROMPT Study). Platelet Receptor Antibodies in Order to Manage Peripheral Artery Thrombosis. *Radiology.* 2001;221:689–696.

90. Yoon HC, Miller FJ, Jr. Using a peptide inhibitor of the glycoprotein IIb/IIIa platelet receptor: initial experience in patients with acute peripheral arterial occlusions. *AJR Am J Roentgenol.* 2002;178:617–622.

91. Visser K, Idu MM, Buth J, Engel GL, Hunink MG. Duplex scan surveillance during the first year after infrainguinal autologous vein bypass grafting surgery: costs and clinical outcomes compared with other surveillance programs. *J Vasc Surg.* 2001;33:123–130.

92. de Vries SO, Visser K, de Vries JA, Wong JB, Donaldson MC, Hunink MG. Intermittent claudication: cost-effectiveness of revascularization versus exercise therapy. *Radiology.* 2002; 222:25–36.

CHAPTER 3
Renal Artery Disease

ANATOMY

The renal arteries and veins typically branch from the aorta and inferior vena cava (IVC), respectively, at the level of the second lumbar vertebral body, below the level of the anterior takeoff of the superior mesenteric artery. The right renal artery passes behind the IVC in its course and is considerably longer than the left renal artery. The main renal artery typically divides into four or more segmental vessels, with five branches most commonly described. The first and most constant segmental division is a posterior branch, which usually exits the main renal artery before it enters the renal hilum and proceeds posteriorly to the renal pelvis to supply a large posterior segment of the kidney. The remaining anterior division of the main renal artery typically branches as it enters the renal hilum. The renal arteries are end branch vessels and do not communicate with each other. This is in contrast to the renal venous system that contains many intrarenal anastomoses.[1] Accessory renal arteries are anatomic variants that occur in 15%–25% of patients.[2]

PATHOPHYSIOLOGY

Table 3.1 summarizes different etiologies of renal artery disease. Renal artery stenosis (RAS) is defined as a greater than 50% narrowing of the renal artery lumen.[3]

Underlying Process

The two most common etiologies of RAS are atherosclerotic renal artery stenosis (ARAS) and fibromuscular dysplasia (FMD).

For ARAS, the underlying pathophysiology involves that of atherosclerotic arterial disease, in general. It is strongly associated with atherosclerotic risk factors, such as diabetes mellitus, dyslipidemia, and smoking.[4, 5]

In cases of FMD involving the renal arteries, the most common histological finding (90% of cases) is that of fibroplasia of the media of the vessel. Other less common histological findings include fibroplasia of the intima or the adventitia. Smoking has been associated with an increased risk for the development of FMD.[5, 6] Table 3.2 provides a classification of the different types of FMD.

Common Pathway: Renin-Angiotensin-Aldosterone System Activation

Despite etiologic differences, all forms of RAS result in a common pathophysiologic pathway that explains the clinical syndromes through which they manifest clinically: The activation of the renin-angiotensin-aldosterone system (RAAS).

Table 3.1   Etiologic Entities Causing Renal Artery Disease

Atherosclerosis
Fibromuscular dysplasia
Post-transplant (site of vascular anastomoses)
Renal artery aneurysm
Takayasu's arteritis
Atheroemboli
Thromboemboli
William's syndrome
Neurofibromatosis
Spontaneous renal artery dissection
Arteriovenous malformations
Arteriovenous fistulae
Trauma
Abdominal radiation therapy
Retroperitoneal fibrosis
External compression from aortic dissection or hematoma

Table 3.2   Classification of Fibromuscular Dysplasia

Classification	Frequency (%)	Pathology	Angiographic Appearance
Medial dysplasia			
Medial fibroplasia	80	Alternating areas of thinned media and thickened fibromuscular ridges containing collagen; internal elastic membrane may be lost in some areas	"String of beads" appearance in which diameter of "beading" is larger than diameter of artery
Perimedial fibroplasia	10–15	Extensive collagen deposition in outer half of media	"Beading" in which "beads" are smaller than diameter of artery
Medial hyperplasia	1–2	True smooth muscle cell hyperplasia without fibrosis	Concentric smooth stenosis (similar to intimal disease)
Intimal fibroplasia	< 10	Circumferential or eccentric deposition of collagen in the intima; no lipid or inflammatory component; internal elastic lamina fragmented or duplicated	Concentric focal band; long, smooth narrowing
Adventitial (periarterial) fibroplasia	< 1	Dense collagen replaces fibrous tissue of adventitia and may extend into surrounding tissue	Extremely rare. Classic angiographic findings have not been described.

Obtained from reference 7.

When the renal artery lumen diameter is reduced, the RAAS is activated in an attempt to preserve adequate renal perfusion. Its activation causes an increase in systemic vascular resistance and leads to sodium retention. These compensatory mechanisms, however, may eventually fail, leading to worsening kidney function and difficult-to-control hypertension.

In the long term, underperfusion of the kidney caused by blood-flow obstruction produces adaptive changes in the kidney parenchyma, including atrophy of tubular cells, fibrosis of the capillary tuft, and intrarenal arterial medial thickening. In addition to underperfusion, angiotensin II also stimulates fibroblast activity, which may lead to fibrosis in the glomerular tuft and in the tubules.[3, 5, 8–10]

Other pathophysiologic mechanisms include activation of the sympathetic nervous system, abnormalities in endothelial nitric oxide, endothelin release, and increased oxidative stress.[9]

Atherosclerotic renal artery disease usually involves the ostial and proximal third of the renal artery (Figure 3.1). In addition to atherogenesis and endothelial injury, spontaneous or iatrogenic atheroemboli may further deteriorate kidney function.[3, 5]

In contrast, FMD typically involves the distal two-thirds of the main renal artery, as well as secondary and tertiary branches (Figure 3.2).[3, 6]

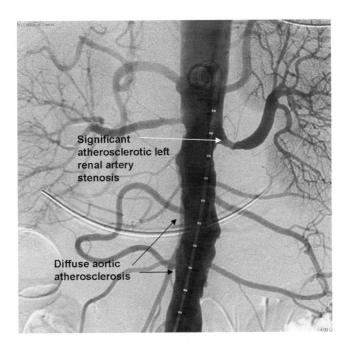

Figure 3.1

Digital substraction angiography in a patient with significant atherosclerotic left renal artery stenosis.

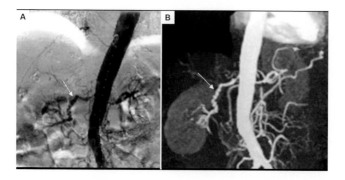

Figure 3.2

Images of a patient with fibromuscular dysplasia of the renal arteries. Panel A: Digital substraction angiography. Panel B: Magnetic Resonance Angiography. Arrows indicate the irregular contour of the dysplastic artery, more evident on the right than on the left.

Figures courtesy of Raul Galvez, MD, MPH and Hale Ersoy, MD; Radiology Department, Brigham and Women's Hospital, Harvard Medical School.

EPIDEMIOLOGY/NATURAL HISTORY

Renal artery stenosis has a prevalence of 0.2%–5% in all hypertensive patients.[8]

Atherosclerosis is the most frequent cause of RAS, accounting for approximately 90% of cases.[3, 11, 12] Its prevalence has been described as high as 25% in patients with coronary artery disease who undergo cardiac catheterization.[5] In the United States, 12%–14% of patients in whom dialysis is initiated have been found to have atherosclerotic RAS.[8, 13] Approximately 2% of the cases of end-stage renal disease are due to the syndrome of ischemic nephropathy.[14]

Fibromuscular dysplasia accounts for 10% of the cases of clinical RAS.[6] It is 2 to 10 times more frequent in females than in males, and these patients are usually diagnosed before the age of 30.[5, 6] The onset of FMD typically occurs before the age of 50.[5, 6]

Renal artery disease is usually progressive in nature and manifests itself as one or more of the clinical syndromes described in the following section. However, even when asymptomatic, it is associated with an increased mortality (Table 3.3). It is also associated with significantly higher cardiovascular event rates (Figure 3.3).

Atherosclerotic RAS is particularly prevalent among individuals with evidence of atherosclerosis in other vascular territories (Table 3.4).

CLINICAL PRESENTATION

RAS often presents as accelerated, resistant, or malignant hypertension. Renal artery stenosis may be associated with acute decline in kidney function after initiation of renin-angiotensin blockade. It may be diagnosed in assessing an unexplained atrophic kidney, or

Table 3.3   Four-Year Survival for Individuals with Incidental (Asymptomatic) RAS as Documented at Cardiac Catheterization

SEVERITY OF INCIDENTAL RAS	FOUR-YEAR SURVIVAL (%)
No RAS	90
50%–75%	70
75%–95%	68
Greater than 95%	48

Adapted from references 5 and 15.

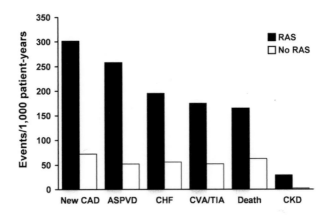

Figure 3.3

Clinical events in patients with RAS. New clinical events reflected as Medicare claims in the 2 years after identification of new atherosclerotic renal artery stenosis (RAS), based on a review of 1,085,250 claims between 1997 and 2001. These observations confirm the increased rate of new cardiovascular events, including death, in patients with identified renovascular disease in the population above age 65 years in the U.S. Cardiovascular events were far more frequent than further loss of kidney function (CKD). ASPVD, atherosclerotic peripheral vascular disease; CAD, coronary artery disease; CHF, congestive heart failure; CKD, chronic kidney disease; CVA, cerebrovascular accident; Dx, diagnosis; TIA, transient ischemic attack.

Reprinted from: JACC Cardiovasc Interv, Vol. 2, McKusick M, Lerman L, Textor S. The uncertain value of renal artery interventions: where are we now?, Page 175, Copyright, 2009, with permission from Elsevier.

discrepancy in kidney size > 1.5 cm or sudden, unexplained, and/or recurrent pulmonary edema. Table 3.5 and Figure 3.4 show certain clinical characteristics of RAS and its two more common etiologies.

The most common diagnoses to be considered in the differential of RAS are provided below in Table 3.6.

Table 3.4   Prevalence of RAS in Individuals with Systemic Atherosclerotic Syndromes

	Abdominal aortic aneurysm (N = 108)	Aortic occlusive disease (N = 21)	Infrainguinal peripheral arterial disease (N = 189)
All patients with greater than 50% stenosis	41 (38%)	7 (33%)	74 (39%)

*p < 0.01 versus other 3 groups. Adapted from references 5 and 16.

Table 3.5   Clinical Characteristics of RAS

CLINICAL SYNDROME	COMMENTS
Hypertension	• Accelerated, malignant, or resistant; patients with RAS can present with severe, progressive, and/or difficult-to-control hypertension, sometimes causing end-organ damage • Hypertension onset before age 30 years suggests FMD • Hypertension onset after age 55 years suggests atherosclerotic RAS
Kidney dysfunction or acute kidney injury	• Unexplained kidney dysfunction may result from progressive stenosis (ischemic nephropathy, atheroemboli, or hypertension-related end-organ damage) • Acute kidney injury can be seen in some patients with bilateral RAS or RAS of a single functioning kidney after starting an ACE inhibitor or ARB
Unexplained congestive heart failure and recurrent pulmonary edema	• Systolic and diastolic heart failure associated with accelerated or difficult-to-control hypertension
Refractory angina	• Usually in association with severe hypertension; concomitant CAD
Absence of family history of hypertension	• May be suggestive of RAS as a cause for hypertension

Key: RAS, renal artery stenosis; FMD, fibromuscular dysplasia; ACE, angiotensin-converting enzyme; ARB, aldosterone receptor blocker; CAD, coronary artery disease. Adapted from references 4, 5, and 8.

DIAGNOSTIC EVALUATION

The evaluation of RAS includes consideration of factors in the history and physical, and decisions regarding appropriate laboratory evaluation and imaging modalities.[17]

In addition to the presence of hypertension and age of onset, the presence of an abdominal bruit should raise the suspicion of the presence of RAS.[5, 8, 18] Bruits in other

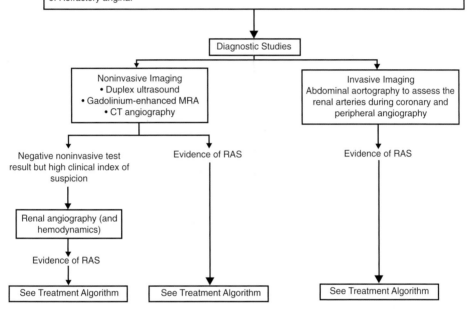

Figure 3.4

Clinical clues to the diagnosis of renal artery stenosis. †For example, atrophic kidney due to chronic pyelonephritis is not an indication for RAS evaluation. ACE, angiotensin-converting enzyme; ARB, angiotensin receptor blocker; CT, computed tomography; LOE, level of evidence; MRA, magnetic resonance angiography.

Reproduced from: Hirsch AT, Haskal ZJ, Hertzer NR, et al. ACC/AHA 2005 Practice Guidelines for the management of patients with peripheral arterial disease. Circulation 2006;113:e463–e654, with the permission of the American Heart Association, Inc.

Table 3.6 Differential Diagnosis of RAS

CLINICAL ENTITY	COMMENTS	EVALUATION
Essential hypertension	Most frequent cause of HTN	Blood pressure measurement, EKG, urinalysis, fundoscopic examination
Acute kidney injury due to other causes	e.g., glomerulopathies	Urine and serum studies; GFR estimation

Continues

Table 3.6   Differential Diagnosis of RAS (Continued)

CLINICAL ENTITY	COMMENTS	EVALUATION
Renal artery dissection	Although FMD places patients at a higher risk of renal artery dissection, primary spontaneous dissection of the renal artery or the aorta (involving the renal arteries) may cause severe hypertension and loss of kidney function	Ultrasound, MRA, CT-angiography, or conventional angiography
Renal artery embolism	History of other vascular disease; history of catheterization (although it may occur spontaneously)	Systemic eosinophilia; urinalysis and sediment evaluation (white blood cells, eosinophils)
Chronic kidney disease, diabetic nephropathy, hypertensive nephrosclerosis	Patients with chronic kidney disease typically have difficult-to-control hypertension and volume status, and may mimic RAS; furthermore, diabetes and hypertension are both causes of CKD as well as RAS	GFR estimation, urinalysis and sediment evaluation, kidney biopsy
Coarctation of the aorta	Can cause misleading and discrepant blood pressure readings	Blood pressure in both arms and legs, echocardiography, MRI, aortography
Primary hyperaldosteronism	Resistant or accelerated hypertension, adrenal adenoma	Plasma and urine potassium, plasma aldosterone to renin ratio > 20 (more specific if > 50), adrenal CT, urine aldosterone after oral salt load, adrenal venous sampling
Cushing syndrome	Moon fascies, buffalo hump, obesity, abdominal striae, possibly history of steroid administration	Morning plasma cortisol after 1 mg dexamethasone at bedtime, urinary cortisol, adrenal CT, scintigrams
Pheochromocytoma	Resistant or accelerated hypertension, possibly episodic hypertension	Plasma-free metanephrines, urine metanephrines and catecholamines, plasma normetanephrine, adrenal CT, scintigrams
Vasculitis	Usually with systemic symptoms (e.g., fever, weight loss), progressive kidney failure	Decreased GFR, abnormal urinalysis and sediment; imaging studies may help

Key: HTN, hypertension; EKG, electrocardiogram; GFR, glomerular filtration rate; FMD, fibromuscular dysplasia; MRA, magnetic resonance angiography; CT, computed tomography; WBC, white blood cells; CKD, chronic kidney disease; RAS, renal artery stenosis.

Table 3.7   General Investigations in Patients with Suspected RAS

INVESTIGATION	COMMENTS
Blood pressure measurement	RAS typically causes clinical hypertension
Serum Creatinine (to estimate GFR)	To estimate the glomerular filtration rate as part of the assessment of kidney function
Serum Potassium	Hypokalemia or low-normal potassium may suggest activation of the renin-angiotensin-aldosterone system
Urine sodium	Low urine sodium may reflect underperfusion of the kidney
Urinalysis and sediment evaluation	To exclude glomerular disease–RAS, in the absence of coexistent diabetic nephropathy or hypertensive nephrosclerosis, is typically non-proteinuric without abnormalities in the urinary sediment
Other evaluation of secondary causes of hypertension as indicated	E.g., an aldosterone to renin ratio < 20 excludes primary hyperaldosteronism
If vasculitis suspected, specific antibodies or cytokine measurements	

Key: GFR, glomerular filtration rate. RAS, renal artery stenosis; Adapted from references 3, 4, 8, 19, and 20.

vessels are frequent due to the common pathophysiology and high prevalence of coexistent peripheral vascular disease.[4]

There is no evidence that screening tests for RAS are useful in the general population. Auscultation for abdominal bruits, however, is advised in the initial evaluation of all hypertensive patients.[18]

A diagnostic evaluation to identify RAS is indicated in patients with hypertension onset before age 30; those with severe hypertension; accelerated hypertension; resistant hypertension; malignant hypertension with acute end-organ damage (acute kidney injury, CHF, neurological disturbance, retinopathy); azotemia after administration of angiotensin converting enzyme (ACE) inhibitor or angiotensin receptor blocker (ARB); unexplained atrophic kidney or a discrepancy in size between the 2 kidneys of greater than 1.5 cm; and sudden unexplained pulmonary edema.

Table 3.7 provides recommendations for general laboratory investigations in patients with suspected RAS.

In addition to basic laboratory data, controversy remains as to what imaging modality is most appropriate. While ultrasonography offers a safe, non-invasive assessment, sensitivity and specificity are lower, evaluations are highly operator dependent, and its use provides only indirect evidence of the presence of stenosis (Figure 3.5). Other non-invasive techniques (i.e., MRA or CT angiography) have risk associated with the use of contrast media (radiocontrast nephropathy and nephrogenic systemic fibrosis, respectively) (Figures 3.6 and 3.7).

Conventional angiography, despite its procedural vascular risks (atheroemboli, bleeding, etc.) and the risk of radiocontrast nephropathy, provides the ability to measure the pressure gradient across a stenotic lesion, and the possibility of concurrently performing endovascular therapy (Figure 3.8).

It has been suggested to start the evaluation of patients with intermediate probability of RAS with a non-invasive imaging test (Table 3.8), and invasive imaging in those with a high probability (Table 3.9).

THERAPEUTIC CONSIDERATIONS

Medical Treatment of RAS

Antihypertensive medications

The majority of patients with RAS have refractory or difficult-to-control hypertension, regardless of the etiology (FMD vs. atherosclerotic). Thus, the first-line treatment for this

Table 3.8   Non-Invasive Imaging Modalities in RAS

Imaging Modality	Comments
Duplex ultrasound (Figure 3.5)	• Sensitivity 84%–98% • Specificity 62%–99% • Can identify discrepancy in kidney size, velocity of renal blood flow, and resistive index[3, 5, 19–21]
Gadolinium-enhanced magnetic resonance angiography (Figure 3.6)	• Sensitivity 90%–100% • Specificity 76%–94% • Visualizes the renal arteries and perirenal aorta[3, 5, 19, 20]
Computed tomography angiography (Figure 3.7)	• Sensitivity 59%–96% • Specificity 82%–99% • Visualizes the renal arteries and perirenal aorta[3, 5, 10, 19, 20]
Captopril renal scan	• Sensitivity 45%–94% • Specificity 81%–100% • Positive if: a) delayed time to maximal radiotracer activity (TMax greater than or equal to 11 minutes after captopril administration), b) significant asymmetry of peak activity of each kidney, c) marked cortical retention of the radionuclide after captopril administration, and d) marked reduction in calculated GFR of the ipsilateral kidney after ACE inhibition • Helpful to assess differential renal flow and kidney function between the two kidneys • Useful in unilateral RAS, but limited in bilateral disease[3, 5, 11, 19, 20]

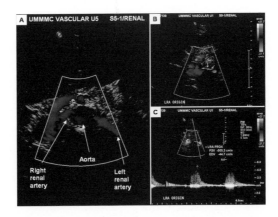

Figure 3.5

Renal duplex ultrasound. Panel A: Normal two-dimensional and color Doppler transverse view of the aorta at the origin of the renal arteries with non-turbulent flow. Panel B: Two-dimensional and color Doppler transverse view of the left renal artery in a patient with significant atherosclerotic renal artery stenosis; arrows indicate heavily calcified plaque in the proximal segment. Panel C: Color and spectral Doppler of the left renal artery show an increased velocity of 50 meters per second in the proximal left renal artery, consistent with severe renal artery stenosis. **See Plate 4 for color image**.

Images courtesy of Denise Kush, RDMS, RVT; Vascular Laboratory, UMass Memorial Health Care.

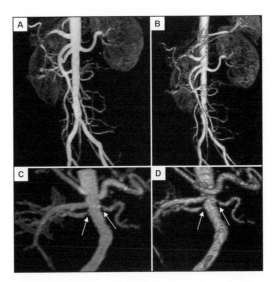

Figure 3.6

Magnetic resonance angiography of the renal arteries. Panels A and B: Normal renal arteries in a two-dimensional maximum intensity projection (MIP) view and a three-dimensional volume rendered reconstruction, respectively. Panels C and D: Bilateral renal artery stenosis (arrows) in a two-dimensional MIP view and a three-dimensional volume rendered reconstruction, respectively.

Figures courtesy of David J. Sheehan, DO; Radiology Department, University of Massachusetts Medical Center and Medical School.

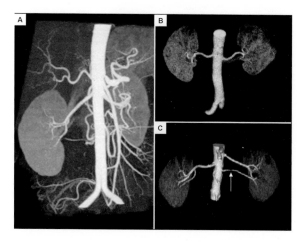

Figure 3.7

Computed tomography angiography of the renal arteries. Panel A: Maximal intensity projection of the aorta and its branches depicts clearly the course of the renal arteries. Panel B: Volume rendered three-dimensional reconstruction in a patient with normal renal arteries. Panel C: Volume rendered three-dimensional reconstruction in a patient with an accessory left renal artery (arrow).

Panel A courtesy of Raul Galvez, MD, MPH and Hale Ersoy, MD; Radiology Department, Brigham and Women's Hospital, Harvard Medical School. Panels B and C courtesy of David J. Sheehan, DO; Radiology Department, University of Massachusetts Medical Center and Medical School.

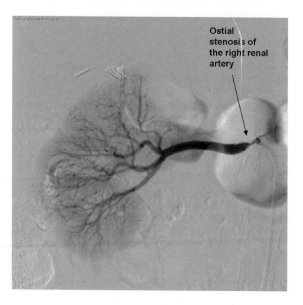

Figure 3.8

Selective angiogram reveals marked ostial stenosis of the right renal artery.

Table 3.9 Invasive Testing Modalities in RAS

IMAGING MODALITY	COMMENTS
Angiography (Figure 3.8)	• Angiography is the gold standard in the evaluation of RAS • Reasonable as first diagnostic test in patients with multivessel coronary artery disease; refractory CHF or refractory angina • Possibility of performing intervention during the procedure • Can measure pressure gradients across stenotic lesion to determine significance: a functional flow reserve < 0.9 as measured by pressure wire across stenotic lesion is considered significant,[22] as is a peak gradient ≥ 20 mmHg or a mean gradient ≥ 10 mmHg (measured with a ≤ 5-Fr catheter or pressure wire) across a stenotic lesion in the renal artery [3, 5, 17, 19, 20]
Selective renal vein renin activity	• Based on unilateral elevation of renin activity on the side of a hemodynamically significant stenosis, although lateralization indices are highly variable and highly controversial[5, 23] • One study showed that if there was lateralization of the renal vein renin ratio of more than 1.4:1 and duration of hypertension less than 5 years, the cure rate of hypertension after revascularization was 95%[24] • Renal vein renin measurements may have more utility in establishing an indication for nephrectomy in patients with renal artery occlusion than in identifying patients with RAS who may derive benefit from revascularization; for pediatric patients with questionably severe RAS before revascularization; or for patients with very marked aortoiliac-renal atherosclerosis, in whom revascularization could carry unusually high risk[5] • Another study showed that lateralization indices did not predict an effect of revascularization, but a peripheral renin concentration lower than 8 mIU/l predicted no effect of intervention[23]

Key: RAS, renal artery stenosis; CHF, congestive heart failure.

condition is blood pressure control to a target of < 130/80 given the high likelihood of concomitant cardiovascular disease (according to the goals of the Seventh Report of the Joint National Committee on Prevention, Detection, Evaluation, and Treatment of High Blood Pressure and according to clinical judgment).[18]

Many patients may already be on antihypertensive medications. Although no data support the use of a single agent or combination of drugs in RAS, the presence of compelling indications for treatment of comorbid conditions makes antihypertensive selection important. Furthermore, combination therapy with multiple agents is often necessary to achieve blood pressure goals.

Only blood pressure control with medications and/or intervention will prevent or limit end-organ damage, such as progression of chronic kidney disease (CKD), and will palliate some of the manifestations of RAS, like refractory pulmonary edema and refractory angina. It is important to consider that patients with atherosclerotic RAS usually have concomitant cardiovascular disease that should be aggressively treated.

Renin-angiotensin blockade with ACE inhibitors or with ARBs are an attractive first-line antihypertensive strategy, as their action targets the mechanism of hypertension in RAS. As hypertension is a consequence of angiotensin II increasing systemic vascular resistance and stimulating sodium retention, ACE inhibitors have the potential to correct this state. However, some patients may not tolerate renin-angiotensin blockade since GFR preservation may be dependent on high angiotensin II effects at the efferent arteriole to maintain intraglomerular pressure. It is recommended that blood pressure, kidney

Table 3.10   Medications and Doses in RAS Trials

ACE inhibitors
Captopril 12.5 mg PO tid to 25 mg PO tid[25, 26]
Enalapril 10–20 mg PO daily[26–28]
Thiazides
HCTZ 25 mg PO daily[27]
Clorothiazide
Bedrofluazide[29]
Loop diuretics
Furosemide 40 mg PO daily[27]
Beta-blockers
Atenolol 50–100 mg PO daily[28, 29]
Calcium channel blockers
Amlodipine 10 mg PO daily[30]
Nifedipine SR 20 mg PO bid[27]
Alpha-antagonists
Prazosin 2.5 mg PO daily[27]
Centrally acting agents
Clonidine 0.15 mg PO bid[27]
Vasodilators
Hydralazine
Other
Methyldopa[29]
Minoxidil

Key: bid, twice daily; tid, three times a day; SR, sustained release; PO, per os (by mouth); HCTZ, hydrochlorothiazide.

Doses (where available) are those of the clinical trials, but certain medications could be uptitrated to much higher doses.

function, and electrolytes be followed closely after initiating therapy. ARBs and direct renin inhibitors have not been studied in this population but are generally considered equivalent to ACE inhibitors.

Table 3.10 outlines medications that have been evaluated in RAS trials. These medications and doses (when available) are not intended to be a guideline for treatment but are only reflective of what was studied in these trials.

Statins

Because atherosclerotic RAS is a type of vascular disease, statins should be considered for all patients. Although direct evidence is lacking for this recommendation, the high prevalence of concomitant peripheral and coronary artery disease makes this recommendation reasonable. However, there are no published studies evaluating particular statin drugs, doses, or LDL cholesterol targets in this population. Weak evidence suggests that statins in general may slow the progression of atherosclerotic RAS.[31, 32] There are no data on the effect of statins on FMD.

Glycemic control

Tight glucose control with a goal HgbA1C < 7% has been shown to decrease cardiovascular mortality in patients with established coronary disease or coronary disease equivalents (i.e., diabetes, peripheral vascular disease).[33] It is known to decrease the risk of microvascular complications and possibly decrease the risk of macrovascular complications.[33, 34] Based on these findings, glucose control is desirable in patients with ARAS.

Antiplatelet therapy

Although antiplatelet therapy has not been studied in patients with RAS, the guidelines suggest consideration of aspirin for all patients with ARAS, due to concomitant coronary and other vascular disease. It is unclear if ASA provides any benefit in patients with FMD.[5, 27, 32]

Lifestyle modifications

A low-salt diet, physical activity, and weight reduction may help improve blood pressure in some patients. Smoking cessation is an important part of the management in both atherosclerotic and FMD RAS patients.[5, 6]

Interventional Treatment of RAS

Figure 3.9 below provides an algorithm for the consideration of an interventional approach in patients with RAS.

Percutaneous treatment of RAS

The preferred treatment modalities differ for patients with FMD or ARAS.

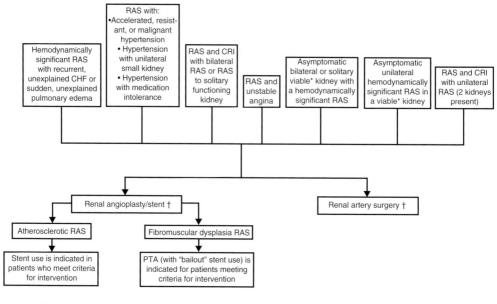

Figure 3.9

Indications for renal revascularization. *Viable means kidney linear length greater than 7 cm. †It is recognized that renal artery surgery has proven efficacy in alleviating RAS due to atherosclerosis and fibromuscular dysplasia. Currently, however, its role is often reserved for individuals in whom less invasive percutaneous RAS interventions are not feasible. CHF, congestive heart failure; CRI, chronic renal insufficiency; LOE, level of evidence; PTA, percutaneous transluminal angioplasty.

Fibromuscular dysplasia   Angioplasty should be considered first-line therapy for FMD, as it is often curative. Angioplasty has an initial technical success of about 90%, and 5- to 10-year patency rates of approximately 85%–90%[35, 36]

Stenting is not indicated for the initial treatment of RAS due to FMD except in cases of procedural complications during percutaneous renal artery balloon angioplasty (i.e., renal artery dissection). Stenting could be considered in the setting of restenosis.[5]

Atherosclerotic RAS   Percutaneous intervention should be considered in patients with difficult-to-control hypertension or end-organ damage despite aggressive medical therapy, in the presence of test results confirmatory of the presence of RAS, as outlined in Table 3.11. There are no data supporting renal artery stenting in asymptomatic patients in whom RAS is incidentally found.[5, 9]

Figures 3.10 and 3.11 depict angiograms prior to and after stenting in a patient with ARAS.

Table 3.11   Conditions in Which Renal Artery Stenting Should be Considered

Refractory hypertension on a multidrug regimen (> 3 medications)
Progressive CKD
AKI on ACE inhibitors/ARBs in patients with CHF
Recurrent flash pulmonary edema
Bilateral renal artery stenosis
Stenosis of renal artery supplying single functioning kidney
Salvage therapy in recent-onset end-stage renal failure
Patients with RAS, uncontrolled hypertension, and unstable angina

Adapted from reference 5. Key: CKD, chronic kidney disease; AKI, acute kidney injury; ACE, angiotensin-converting enzyme; ARB, angiotensin receptor blockers; CHF, congestive heart failure; RAS, renal artery stenosis.

Treatment considerations are difficult in this population. A recent systematic review for the Agency for Healthcare Research and Quality aimed at comparing the effects of medical treatment and revascularization on clinically important outcomes in adults with ARAS found no trials comparing aggressive medical therapy and angioplasty with stent placement. In this review, some evidence suggested similar kidney outcomes but better blood pressure outcomes with balloon angioplasty alone, particularly in patients with bilateral renal disease. Weak evidence suggested no large differences in mortality or cardiovascular events between medical and revascularization treatments. There was no direct comparison of adverse event rates between different treatment modalities. Furthermore, many of the studies were outdated and did not reflect current clinical practice (i.e., renal artery stenting).[13] Table 3.12 summarizes the findings of this review.

The results of the Angioplasty and Stenting for Renal Artery Lesions (ASTRAL) study were recently presented. It included patients with significant ARAS, who were randomized to angioplasty and/or stenting plus medical therapy (n = 403; 93% received stents) or medical therapy alone (n = 403). The primary endpoint was kidney function, measured by the reciprocal of the serum creatinine. The stenting group had a slower decline in kidney function at 5-year follow up, but this benefit appeared to be offset by procedural complications. Similarly, the STAR trial randomized 140 patients with ARAS to stent placement plus medical therapy versus medical therapy (antihypertensive therapy, aspirin, and a statin). The primary endpoint was a $\geq 20\%$ decrease in creatinine clearance. The primary endpoint was reached by 16% in the stent group and 22% in the medical therapy group (p = ns). However, these two trials were limited by imprecise definitions of RAS, inclusion of patients with clinically insignificant lesions, crossovers, and inadequately specified medical interventions. In addition, these trials evaluated surrogate end points such as kidney function and blood pressure, and they were not powered to assess differences in cardiovascular event rates.[37, 40]

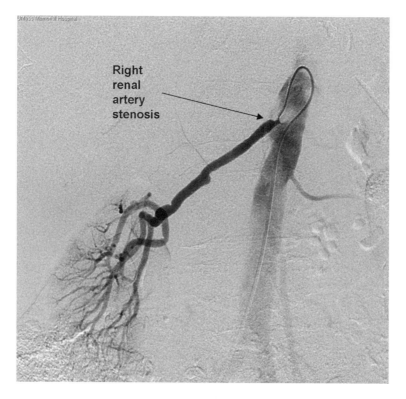

Figure 3.10

Selective angiogram reveals marked ostial stenosis of the right renal artery.

The ongoing Cardiovascular Outcomes in Renal Atherosclerotic Lesions (CORAL) trial is enrolling patients with atherosclerotic renal artery stenosis with at least 60% stenosis and systolic hypertension for which they are receiving two or more antihypertensive medications. Patients with advanced chronic kidney disease (serum creatinine concentration > 3.0 mg/dL), those with very small kidneys, and certain patients with cardiovascular disease are being excluded. This trial will address many of the deficiencies in current evidence about revascularization plus medical therapy versus medical therapy alone.[38]

Surgical treatment of RAS

Renal artery surgery has proven efficacy in alleviating RAS due to both ARAS and FMD. However, the current role of surgery is often reserved for individuals in whom less invasive percutaneous RAS interventions are not feasible or for individuals undergoing concomitant surgical repair of the abdominal aorta (e.g., aneurysm). As mentioned

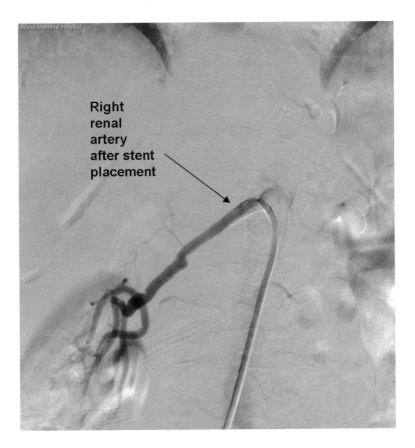

Right
renal
artery
after stent
placement

Figure 3.11

Selective angiogram reveals excellent angiographic result after right renal artery stenting.

above, for patients with ARAS, there is no evidence to support medical therapy alone versus percutaneous or surgical intervention. The decision to perform surgical renal revascularization should be made on an individual basis.[5]

CONTROVERSIES AND FUTURE DIRECTIONS

Although RAS is associated with an overall decreased survival and kidney outcomes, the heterogeneity in its etiology, clinical manifestations, treatment approaches, and outcomes has sparked a debate as to how to better define it (and its comorbidities) and how to select patients better. Tables 3.13 and 3.14 summarize some recommendations that may shape future clinical management and research in RAS.

Table 3.12   Effects of Renal Artery Revascularization versus Medical Treatment Alone on Clinical Outcomes

Outcomes	Strength of Evidence	Studies (Participants), N			Conclusions
		Randomized Trials	Other Comparative Studies	Cohort Studies	
Death	Weak	1 (55)	4 (381)	30 (4,646)	No large difference in mortality up to about 5 years between revascularization and medical treatment
Kidney function	Acceptable	2 (103)	7 (428)	34 (4,916)	No substantial difference in kidney function; improvements in kidney function were reported in cohort studies only among patients receiving revascularization
Blood pressure	Acceptable	2 (103)	8 (597)	34 (4,275)	Some evidence that blood pressure may be lowered more after angioplasty than with medical treatment alone, particularly among patients with bilateral disease (range, no difference to 26/10 mmHg lower after angioplasty); cure of hypertension was reported in cohort studies only among patients receiving revascularization
Cardiovascular events	Weak	1 (55)	1 (52)	3 (560)	No large differences found in comparative studies up to about 4 years
Adverse events	Weak	2 (103)	4 (323)	31 (4,906)	Evidence does not support meaningful conclusions about relative adverse events or complications from angioplasty compared with medical treatment

Adapted from reference 13.

Table 3.13   Suggested Considerations in the Approach to RAS

Reserve the term "renovascular hypertension" specifically for patients with renin-dependent hypertension, in whom revascularization is expected to cure hypertension. For practical purposes, this is true for most patients with FMD but not all with ARAS.

Hypertension in patients with ARAS might be classified as controlled, refractory, accelerated, or malignant, depending on the clinical circumstances. Patients with ARAS and hypertension should not be classified as having "renovascular hypertension," unless there is evidence that ARAS is the cause of their hypertension.

The term "renal ischemia" should be reserved for patients with RAS and abnormal renal perfusion (unilateral or bilateral).

The term "renal artery stenosis" should be used for patients with "anatomic" stenosis but has no implications regarding renal ischemia.

The term "nephropathy" should be reserved for patients with renal parenchymal disease. "Ischemic nephropathy" should be reserved for patients with renal parenchymal disease associated with long-standing atherosclerosis and intrarenal arteriolar disease. Other forms of nephropathy might be based on the presence of known diseases, such as diabetes (diabetic nephropathy), hypertension (hypertensive nephropathy), or interstitial diseases (interstitial nephropathy) or might be acquired as a complication of revascularization (acute tubular necrosis, contrast nephropathy, and renal embolization).

Medical therapies, particularly antihypertensive drug therapy and therapies to limit ARAS, are the primary therapies for all patients with RAS.

The optimal use of renal artery revascularization is poorly defined. Contemporary decisions about renal revascularization must include an assessment of the severity and functional significance of RAS (renal ischemia), the condition of the kidneys (nephropathy), and the association between RAS and vital organ injury.

The benefits and risks of renal revascularization will be improved by careful patient selection. Better results will be achieved in patients with vital organ injury, renal ischemia, and no nephropathy.

Appropriately designed randomized clinical trials are essential to define the role of renal revascularization. Such trials must incorporate assessment of renal ischemia and nephropathy, because these factors have the strongest influence on outcome.

Table adapted from reference 39.

Table 3.14   Suggested Terminology for Renal Vascular Diseases

Hypertension

- Renovascular hypertension: renin-dependent hypertension, typical of young patients with FMD; characterized by high likelihood of cure of hypertension after revascularization.
- Essential hypertension: typical form of hypertension in elderly persons, associated with manifestations of atherosclerosis; causal relationship between ARAS and hypertension is absent.
- Controlled hypertension: blood pressure controlled with two medications according to current guidelines.
- Refractory hypertension: blood pressure exceeds current guidelines despite three medications.

Continues

Table 3.14   Suggested Terminology for Renal Vascular Diseases (Continued)

- Accelerated hypertension: previously controlled hypertension becomes progressively uncontrolled, exceeds current guidelines, and remains poorly controlled despite multiple additional medications.
- Malignant hypertension: uncontrolled hypertension associated with acute renal or cardiovascular injury.

Renal artery stenosis (no ischemia)

- Unilateral RAS: anatomic unilateral RAS without objective renal ischemia.
- Bilateral RAS: Anatomic bilateral RAS without objective renal ischemia.

Renal ischemia

- Unilateral RAS: objective renal ischemia in the distribution of the stenotic renal artery.
- Bilateral RAS: objective renal ischemia in one or both renal arteries.

Nephropathy (parenchymal disease)

- Ischemic nephropathy: renal parenchymal disease due to long-standing intrarenal arteriolar disease associated with generalized atherosclerosis.
- Diabetic nephropathy: renal parenchymal disease due to long-standing diabetes.
- Hypertensive nephropathy: renal parenchymal disease due to long-standing hypertension, intrarenal arteriolar disease, and self-perpetuating hypertension.
- Other nephropathies: renal parenchymal diseases associated with other known glomerular or interstitial renal diseases.
- Procedure-related nephropathy: acquired parenchymal injury (transient or permanent) that might be related to acute tubular necrosis, radiographic contrast, renal embolization, or other causes.

Table adapted from reference 39.

◇◇◇◇◇◇◇◇◇◇◇◇

REFERENCES

1. Olumi AF, Richie JP. Urologic surgery. In: Townsend CMJ, Beauchamp RD, Evers BM, Mattox KL, eds. *Sabiston Textbook of Surgery: The Biological Basis of Modern Surgical Practice*. 18th ed. Philadelphia, PA: Saunders Elsevier; 2007:2251.

2. Koca N, Ko Z, Kizilkili O, Tercan F, Oguzkurt L, Ozkan U. Renal artery origins and variations: angiographic evaluation of 855 consecutive patients. *Diagnostic and Interventional Radiology*. 2006;12:183.

3. Safian RD, Textor SC. Renal-artery stenosis. *N Engl J Med*. 2001;344:431–442.

4. Eisenhauer AC, White CJ. Endovascular treatment of noncoronary obstructive vascular disease. In: Libby P, Bonow RO, Mann DL, Zipes DP, Braunwald E, eds. *Braunwald's Heart Disease*. 8th ed. Philadelphia, PA: Elsevier Saunders; 2008:1532–1535.

5. Hirsch AT, Haskal ZJ, Hertzer NR, et al. ACC/AHA 2005 Practice Guidelines for the management of patients with peripheral arterial disease (lower extremity, renal, mesenteric, and abdominal aortic): a collaborative report from the American Association for Vascular Surgery/Society for Vascular Surgery, Society for Cardiovascular Angiography and Interventions, Society for Vascular Medicine and Biology, Society of Interventional Radiology, and the ACC/AHA Task Force on Practice Guidelines (Writing Committee to Develop Guidelines for the Management of Patients With Peripheral Arterial Disease): Endorsed by the American Association of Cardiovascular and Pulmonary Rehabilitation; National Heart, Lung, and Blood Institute; Society for Vascular Nursing; TransAtlantic Inter-Society Consensus; and Vascular Disease Foundation. *Circulation*. 2006;113:e463–e654.

6. Slovut DP, Olin JW. Fibromuscular dysplasia. *N Engl J Med*. 2004;350:1862–1871.

7. Olin JW, Begelman SM. Fibromuscular dysplasia. *Curr Opin Rheumatol.* 2000;12:41.

8. Kaplan NM. Renovascular hypertension. In: Kaplan NM, ed. *Clinical Hypertension.* 8th ed. Philadelphia, PA: Lippincott Williams and Wilkins; 2002; 381–403.

9. Haller C, Keim M. Current issues in the diagnosis and management of patients with renal artery stenosis: a cardiologic perspective. *Prog Cardiovasc Dis.* 2003; 46:271–286.

10. Olbricht CJ, Paul K, Prokop M, et al. Minimally invasive diagnosis of renal artery stenosis by spiral computed tomography angiography. *Kidney Int.* 1995;48:1332–1337.

11. Garovic VD, Textor SC. Renovascular hypertension and ischemic nephropathy. *Circulation.* 2005;112:1362–1374.

12. Hansen KJ, Edwards MS, Craven TE, et al. Prevalence of renovascular disease in the elderly: a population-based study. *J Vasc Surg.* 2002;36:443–451.

13. Balk E, Raman G, Chung M, et al. Effectiveness of management strategies for renal artery stenosis: a systematic review. *Ann Intern Med.* 2006;145:901–912.

14. Fatica RA, Port FK, Young EW. Incidence trends and mortality in end-stage renal disease attributed to renovascular disease in the United States. *Am J Kidney Dis.* 2001;37:1184–1190.

15. Mark DB, Pieper K, Little MA, Conlon PJ. Severity of renal vascular disease predicts mortality in patients undergoing coronary angiography. *Kidney Int.* 2001; 60:1490.

16. Risius B, Graor RA, Young JR, Melia M, Olin JW. Prevalence of atherosclerotic renal artery stenosis in patients with atherosclerosis elsewhere. *Am J Med.* 1990;88:46.

17. White CJ. Catheter-based therapy for atherosclerotic renal artery stenosis. *Prog Cardiovasc Dis.* 2007;50: 136–150.

18. Chobanian AV, Bakris GL, Black HR, et al. The Seventh Report of the Joint National Committee on Prevention, Detection, Evaluation, and Treatment of High Blood Pressure: the JNC 7 report. *JAMA.* 2003;289:2560–2572.

19. Chonchol M, Linas S. Diagnosis and management of ischemic nephropathy. *Clin J Am Soc Nephrol.* 2006;1:172–181.

20. Zucchelli PC. Hypertension and atherosclerotic renal artery stenosis: diagnostic approach. *J Am Soc Nephrol.* 2002;13(Suppl 3):S184–S186.

21. Radermacher J. Resistive index: an ideal test for renovascular disease or ischemic nephropathy? *Nat Clin Pract Nephrol.* 2006;2:232–233.

22. Heyndrickx G, Vanderheyden M, Bartunek J, et al. Assessment of renal artery stenosis severity by pressure gradient measurements. *J Am Coll Cardiol.* 2006;48:1851.

23. Hasbak P, Jensen LT, Ibsen H, East Danish Study Group on Renovascular Hypertension. Hypertension and renovascular disease: follow-up on 100 renal vein renin samplings. *J Hum Hypertens.* 2002;16: 275–280.

24. Feinstein AR, Gifford RW, Jr., Dove HG, Hughes JS. Duration of blood pressure elevation in accurately predicting surgical cure of renovascular hypertension. *Am Heart J.* 1981;101:408.

25. Miyamori I, Yasuhara S, Takeda Y, et al. Effects of converting enzyme inhibition on split renal function in renovascular hypertension. *Hypertension.* 1986;8:415–421.

26. Reams GP, Singh A, Logan KW, Holmes RA, Bauer JH. Total and split renal function in patients with renovascular hypertension: effects of angiotensin-converting enzyme inhibition. *J Clin Hypertens.* 1987;3:153–163.

27. Plouin PF, Chatellier G, Darne B, Raynaud A. Blood pressure outcome of angioplasty in atherosclerotic renal artery stenosis: a randomized trial. Essai Multicentrique Medicaments vs Angioplastie (EMMA) Study Group. *Hypertension.* 1998;31:823–829.

28. van Jaarsveld BC, Krijnen P, Pieterman H, et al. The effect of balloon angioplasty on hypertension in atherosclerotic renal-artery stenosis. Dutch Renal Artery Stenosis Intervention Cooperative Study Group. *N Engl J Med.* 2000;342:1007–1014.

29. Webster J, Marshall F, Abdalla M, et al. Randomised comparison of percutaneous angioplasty vs. continued medical therapy for hypertensive patients with atheromatous renal artery stenosis. Scottish and Newcastle Renal Artery Stenosis Collaborative Group. *J Hum Hypertens.* 1998;12:329–335.

30. Krijnen P, van Jaarsveld BC, Deinum J, Steyerberg EW, Habbema JD. Which patients with hypertension and atherosclerotic renal artery stenosis benefit from immediate intervention? *J Hum Hypertens.* 2004;18:91–96.

31. Cheung CM, Patel A, Shaheen N, et al. The effects of statins on the progression of atherosclerotic renovascular disease. *Nephron Clin Pract.* 2007;107:c35–c42.

32. Hanzel G, Balon H, Wong O, Soffer D, Lee DT, Safian RD. Prospective evaluation of aggressive medical therapy for atherosclerotic renal artery stenosis, with renal artery stenting reserved for previously injured heart, brain, or kidney. *Am J Cardiol.* 2005;96:1322–1327.

33. Expert Panel on Detection, Evaluation, and Treatment of High Blood Cholesterol in Adults. Executive summary of the Third Report of The National Cholesterol Education Program (NCEP) Expert Panel on Detection, Evaluation, and Treatment of High Blood Cholesterol in Adults (Adult Treatment Panel III). *JAMA*. 2001;285:2486–2497.

34. UK Prospective Diabetes Study (UKPDS) Group. Intensive blood-glucose control with sulphonylureas or insulin compared with conventional treatment and risk of complications in patients with type 2 diabetes (UKPDS 33). *Lancet.* 1998;352:837–853.

35. Uder M, Humke U. Endovascular therapy of renal artery stenosis: Where do we stand today? *Cardiovasc Intervent Radiol.* 2005;28:139–147.

36. Davies MG, Saad WE, Peden EK, Mohiuddin IT, Naoum JJ, Lumsden AB. The long-term outcomes of percutaneous therapy for renal artery fibromuscular dysplasia. *J Vasc Surg.* 2008;48:865–871.

37. ASTRAL Investigators, Wheatley K, Ives N, et al. Revascularization versus medical therapy for renal-artery stenosis. N Engl J Med. 2009;361:1953–1962.

38. Cooper CJ, Murphy TP, Matsumoto A, et al. Stent revascularization for the prevention of cardiovascular and renal events among patients with renal artery stenosis and systolic hypertension: rationale and design of the CORAL trial. *Am Heart J.* 2006;152:59–66.

39. Madder R, Safian R. Refining the approach to renal artery revascularization. *JACC Cardiovasc Interv.* 2009;2:161.

40. Bax L, Woittiez AJ, Kouwenberg HJ, et al. Stent placement in patients with atherosclerotic renal artery stenosis and impaired renal function: a randomized trial. *Ann Intern Med.* 2009;150:840–848.

CHAPTER 4

Splanchnic and Mesenteric Artery Disease

ANATOMY

Celiac Artery

The celiac artery arises from the ventral surface of the aorta at the level of the T12 or L1 vertebral body. It usually courses anteriorly and slightly inferiorly 1 to 2 cm before branching into the common hepatic, splenic, and left gastric arteries. This classic pattern is observed in 65%–75% of subjects. In 1% or less, there is a common origin of the celiac and superior mesenteric (SMA) branches, a celiacomesenteric trunk.

The splenic artery is one of the three major branches of the celiac axis. The splenic artery arises 1 to 2 cm from the celiac origin and courses to the left in a tortuous path before branching into multiple terminal branches and entering the splenic hilum. Usually the first branch of the splenic artery is the dorsal pancreatic artery, which supplies the posterior or dorsal surface of the pancreas and gives rise to the transverse pancreatic artery to supply the body and tail. The dorsal pancreatic artery also has anastomotic communications with the anterosuperior pancreaticoduodenal and gastroduodenal arteries. The left gastroepiploic artery originates from the splenic artery just before its terminal divisions. It is contained within the omentum and gives rise to the left epiploic artery, which communicates with the right epiploic artery (arising from the right gastroepiploic artery). Multiple short gastric arteries also arise from the distal splenic artery to supply the fundus of the stomach.

The hepatic artery is, in most people, a branch of the celiac artery. However, in 10%–18% of cases, the right hepatic artery takes its origin from the SMA. Great variability is found within the intrahepatic branches. The right hepatic artery supplies the right lobe and usually the caudate lobe of the liver. Supply to the left lobe is from the middle and left hepatic arteries. The left hepatic artery may arise from, or have accessory branches from, the left gastric artery in up to 26% of cases.

The gastroduodenal artery is the first branch of the common hepatic artery in approximately 75% of people. Less commonly, it may arise from the right hepatic artery (7%–10%), the left hepatic artery (10%–12%), or rarely, SMA via a replaced common hepatic artery. The terminal branches of the gastroduodenal artery are the right gastroepiploic artery and the antero- and posterosuperior pancreaticoduodenal arteries. The right gastroepiploic artery communicates with the left gastroepiploic artery arising from the splenic artery in 90% of patients. The posterosuperior pancreaticoduodenal artery is also known as the retroduodenal artery and may arise from the common hepatic or right hepatic arteries. The supraduodenal artery arises either from the retroduodenal artery (50%) or from the gastroduodenal artery (25%) and supplies the proximal duodenum. Both the anterosuperior and the posterosuperior pancreaticoduodenal arteries have anastomotic communications with the corresponding antero- and posteroinferior pancreaticoduodenal arteries arising from the SMA.

The cystic artery arises from the right hepatic artery in 45%–50% of patients, with less common origins from a replaced right hepatic artery from the SMA (10%), from the left or common hepatic arteries (10%), or, uncommonly, from the gastroduodenal artery (< 2%). In 20%–25%, the cystic artery may be duplicated with both branches from the same or two separate right hepatic branches.

The left gastric artery is the third major branch of the celiac artery. It takes its origin from the celiac in more than 90% of people, with 3%–4% arising from the aorta directly. Its posterior division anastomoses with the right gastric artery along the lesser curvature of the stomach.

Accessory left gastric branches may arise from the celiac artery or from the splenic artery. In 12% of patients, the left hepatic artery arises from the left gastric artery, and in an additional 12%–14%, an accessory left hepatic artery arises from the left gastric artery.

Superior Mesenteric Artery

The SMA arises from the aorta approximately 1 cm below the celiac artery, usually at the level of L1. It courses inferiorly and toward the right to terminate at the level of the cecum as the ileocolic artery. The major branches of the SMA include the inferior pancreaticoduodenal artery, the middle colic artery, the right colic artery, 4–6 jejunal branches, and 9–13 branches to the ileum and the ileocolic artery.

The inferior pancreaticoduodenal artery is one of the first branches of the SMA. It arises as two separate branches in 60% of people and as a common trunk in 40% before dividing to form the antero- and posteroinferior pancreaticoduodenal arteries, which anastomose with corresponding superior branches from the celiac axis. Generally there are more SMA branches to the distal small bowel than to the more proximal portions, thus providing greater potential for distal anastomotic communication. The middle colic artery arises from the proximal SMA to supply the transverse colon and communicates with branches of the inferior mesenteric artery (IMA). Multiple variant origins of the middle colic artery have been described, including celiac, SMA, common hepatic, and splenic origins. From the SMA, the middle colic artery may arise from a replaced right or common hepatic artery or from the gastroduodenal artery. The right colic artery arises as a common trunk with the middle colic artery in 50% of cases, with a separate origin from the SMA as the next most common variant (40%). The ileocolic artery is the terminal branch of the SMA and supplies the distal ileum, cecum, and ascending colon. The right and middle colic arteries supply portions of the marginal artery running along the mesenteric side of the colon and also give rise to the terminal vasa recta that provide blood to the colon.

Inferior Mesenteric Artery

The IMA is usually the smallest of the mesenteric vessels and arises from the ventral aorta approximately 6–7 cm below the SMA at the level of L3. It supplies the hindgut including the distal transverse, descending, and sigmoid colon, as well as the rectum. Major branches of the IMA include the left colic, sigmoid, and hemorrhoidal arteries.

The ascending branch of the IMA, or left colic artery, has anastomotic communications with the SMA via the marginal artery, as well as variable additional communications lying within the mesentery. The ascending branch reaches the splenic flexure in 80%–85% of patients and extends to the mid transverse colon in 15%–20%. There is great variability in the blood supply to the splenic flexure, and the middle colic artery may be the predominant or only source of blood to this region. Because, as noted previously, the origin of the middle colic artery may be from branches of the celiac or SMA, supply to the splenic flexure may depend on the integrity of the more proximal vasculature, rather than the more common blood supply from the IMA. Branches to the sigmoid colon may arise from the ascending, middle, or descending branches of the IMA. The superior rectal artery is the distal continuation of the IMA. It commonly divides into two branches; the larger right branch supplies the dorsal and lateral aspects of the rectum, and the left branch generally supplies the ventral aspect of the rectum.

Collateral Flow Patterns

The sources of collateral flow between the mesenteric vessels, as well as between the mesenteric vessels and the non-mesenteric systemic circulation, are numerous. Because of the multiple potential sources of collateral flow, at least two of the three major vessels must be occluded or have critical stenoses for mesenteric ischemia to ensue. Although collaterals may be small or angiographically occult in the non-diseased circulation, they have the potential to markedly increase in size when increased flow is required.[1]

Figures 4.1 to 4.3 depict the normal anatomy of the mesenteric vessels.

PHYSIOLOGY AND PATHOPHYSIOLOGY

Physiology of the Mesenteric Circulation—Vasoreactivity

The mesenteric vessels are among the most reactive in the body. Substantial changes in blood flow are observed with the infusion of multiple classes of pharmacologic agents, including alpha-adrenergic agonists, some prostaglandins and leukotrienes, acetylcholine, serotonin, vasopressin, angiotensin II, somatostatin, digoxin, and endothelin-1 and 3.

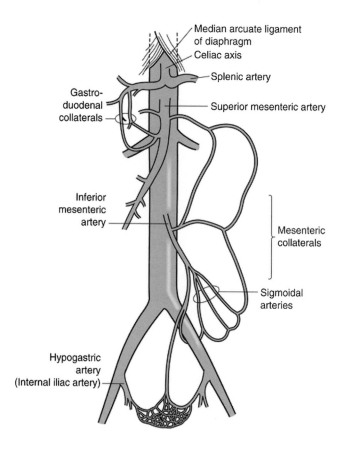

Figure 4.1

Diagram of the mesenteric arterial anatomy demonstrating extensive collateral channels between major branches.

Reproduced with permission from Sabiston textbook of surgery: the biological basis of modern surgical practice. 18th ed. Philadelphia, PA: Saunders Elsevier, 2007:1974.

This hyperreactivity of the splanchnic vessels accounts, in part, for the wide fluctuations in blood flow observed between fasting and food ingestion, as well as during non-occlusive ischemia and vasospasm.

Physiology of the Mesenteric Circulation—Splanchnic Blood Flow

Splanchnic blood flow can fluctuate between 10% and 35% of cardiac output depending on the magnitude, time, and composition of food ingestion. Absolute measurements of mean blood flow in the revascularized human celiac axis and SMA vary from 300 to 1200 mL/min. These values are among the highest for any type of bypass graft. At rest, the mesenteric outflow bed exhibits intermediate to high resistance with low

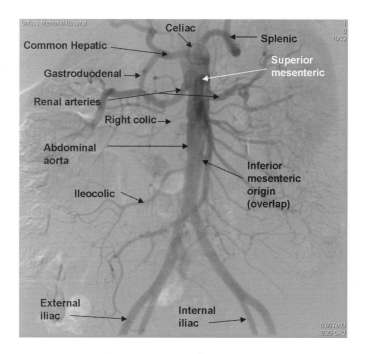

Figure 4.2

Digital substraction angiography of abdominal and mesenteric vessels.

diastolic flow and a component of flow reversal. With nutrition, antegrade flow is observed throughout the cardiac cycle, typical of maximally dilated, low-resistance beds.

The capacity of the splanchnic bed to widely vary its blood flow is thought to arise from multiple levels of local and regional control. Control mechanisms can be classified into intrinsic and extrinsic systems. Intrinsic regulation of mesenteric blood flow occurs through metabolic and myogenic pathways. Metabolic regulation occurs as the by-products of mucosal ischemia (e.g., adenosine) exert a direct vasorelaxant effect on arteriolar smooth muscle, enhancing whole organ perfusion as well as preferentially redistributing flow to the mucosa. Smooth muscle cell relaxation can also be induced by a decrease in perfusion pressure, probably as a result of local release of nitric oxide. These mechanisms account for the phenomenon of blood flow autoregulation or the ability to preserve mucosal oxygen delivery in the setting of systemic hypotension. Intestinal blood flow is also controlled extrinsically through neural and hormonal axes.[1]

All diseases and conditions that affect arteries have been reported in the arteries that supply the intestines, including atherosclerosis, arteritis, aneurysms, arterial infections, fibromuscular dysplasia, dissections, arterial emboli, and thrombosis.[2] Mesenteric ischemia occurs when visceral tissues receive inadequate blood flow. This may be a consequence

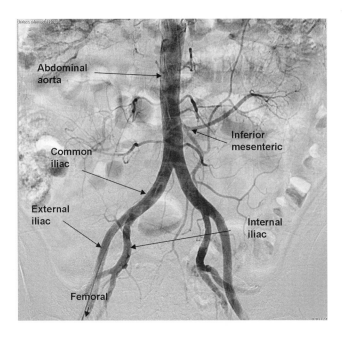

Figure 4.3

Digital substraction angiography shows in greater detail the course of the inferior mesenteric artery.

of an arterial embolus or thrombosis, venous thrombosis limiting arterial inflow, or even extrinsic compression of mesenteric vessels. When demand exceeds the capacity of the mesenteric circulation because of intrinsic or extrinsic lesions, the bowel becomes ischemic, with the mucosa being most vulnerable to inadequate blood flow. When the integrity of the bowel wall is disrupted, there may be translocation of bacteria, which may lead to endotoxemia and eventually septic shock. When necrosis ensues, there is extravasation of the bowel contents into the peritoneal cavity, leading to peritonitis and sepsis.

Mesenteric arterial thrombosis often occurs in patients with prior progressive atherosclerotic stenoses, with superimposed abdominal trauma or infection. Mesenteric venous thrombosis, however, may occur in the setting of hypercoagulable states, blunt trauma, abdominal infection, portal hypertension, pancreatitis, or malignancy.

EPIDEMIOLOGY/NATURAL HISTORY

Mesenteric ischemia accounts for fewer than 1 in every 1000 hospital admissions,[3] but is a highly morbid condition. Mortality rates are 30%–90%, depending on the etiology.[4, 5]

Its difficult diagnosis may account in part for the high morbidity and mortality. In one review, only one-third of patients who had acute mesenteric ischemia were correctly diagnosed before surgical exploration or death.[6] Similarly, in an autopsy series, in only 33% of patients whose cause of death was determined to be mesenteric ischemia was the diagnosis considered.[7]

It is important to stratify mesenteric artery disease based on its etiology.

Approximately two-thirds of patients with acute intestinal ischemia are women, with a median age of 70 years.[2]

Embolism

Embolism to the visceral vessels is the most common cause of mesenteric ischemia, responsible for approximately 30%–50% of cases.[8, 9]

Risk factors for visceral emboli include atrial fibrillation, myocardial infarction, valvular heart disease, endocarditis, and structural heart defects. Catheterization (cardiac or peripheral) with passage of catheters into the aorta is another important risk factor. The acuity of presentation, combined with frequent delays in the diagnosis, contribute to a high mortality rate, which averages 70%.[4]

Thrombosis

Thrombosis of arterial mesenteric inflow accounts for only 15%–30% of cases of mesenteric ischemia. It carries, however, the highest mortality rate, 90%.[4] This high mortality rate has been hypothesized to be a consequence of plaque rupture and subsequent thrombosis in the more proximal portion of the mesenteric vessel, thus affecting a greater percentage of the overall bowel.

Non-occlusive Ischemia

Non-occlusive ischemia is nearly always due to atherosclerosis, either from functional mismatch between oxygen supply and demand, or from a consequence of low-flow states. The majority of patients (75%) are smokers. In contrast to other vascular syndromes, approximately 60% of patients are female. More than one-third of patients have hypertension, coronary artery disease, and/or cerebrovascular disease. About 20% have evidence of chronic kidney disease, and many are diabetics.[10]

Acute non-occlusive mesenteric ischemia usually occurs in the setting of atherosclerotic vascular disease, oftentimes in a patient with an acute cardiovascular disease process who is being treated with drugs that reduce intestinal perfusion. This may include patients with recent cardiac surgery, and dialysis patients. Cocaine use has also been a causative factor in a number of cases.

Chronic non-occlusive ischemia affects women more frequently, for reasons that are not completely understood. These patients usually have other atherosclerotic risk factors. Although the prevalence of splanchnic and mesenteric atherosclerosis is between

30% and 50% in autopsy series, only a small portion of patients develop the syndrome of intestinal angina.[10]

A less frequent cause of non-occlusive ischemia is extrinsic compression of the celiac artery (arcuate ligament syndrome, also referred to as celiac compression syndrome). It results from impingement of the diaphragm and the celiac nerve plexus on the celiac artery. It occurs more frequently in younger women.[10]

Finally, liver transplant recipients can also experience stenosis of the anastomosed celiac artery.[11]

Venous Thrombosis

Venous thrombosis accounts for a minority of cases of disease of the mesenteric circulation but is associated with a mortality rate between 20% and 50%.[5] Most cases are associated with cirrhosis or portal hypertension. Other etiologies include malignancy, pancreatitis, oral contraceptive use, inheritable hypercoagulable states, or a history of recent surgery.[5, 9] Half of patients presenting with venous thrombosis have had a deep venous thrombosis or pulmonary embolus in the past.[5]

CLINICAL PRESENTATION AND PHYSICAL EXAM

Mesenteric and splanchnic disease are challenging to diagnose. Patients most often present with vague abdominal pain. Other associated symptoms, such as nausea, vomiting, diarrhea, and bloating, may also be present. The typical non-specific presentation usually leads to delays in the diagnosis and treatment.

Embolic

Patients with embolic disease usually present with acute and rapid progression of symptoms. The typical patient who has visceral ischemia from an embolic source reports the sudden onset of severe pain. Physical examination is often notable for the lack of guarding or peritoneal signs, so-called "pain out of proportion" to examination. Peritoneal findings may occur late, following embolic occurrences, after the development of infarcted bowel, and typically portend worse outcomes. The SMA is more commonly involved than the celiac axis (CA) or IMA because of its less acute angle of takeoff from the aorta. Emboli typically lodge distal to the takeoff of the middle colic artery, sparing the duodenum and the transverse colon—a characteristic that can often help differentiate it from thrombosis that typically occurs more proximally.[12, 13]

Thrombotic

The presentation of acute mesenteric thrombosis is similar to that of acute embolism. However, most patients suffering from acute mesenteric arterial thrombosis have a history of chronic mesenteric ischemia, with symptoms of weight loss, abdominal pain, and food fear (see below).

Non-occlusive Ischemia or Chronic Mesenteric Ischemia

Patients who have chronic mesenteric ischemia typically present with postprandial abdominal pain and associated weight loss. This pain occurs within the first hour after eating and diminishes 1–2 hours later. The postprandial timing of the pain is most directly attributed to the limitation in blood flow through the celiac and SMA lesions in the face of increased metabolic demands after a meal. Others have suggested that the ischemia is actually caused by a steal phenomenon from the intestinal to the gastric circulation when food is introduced into the stomach, better explaining the temporal nature of the pain. Postprandial symptoms usually require occlusion of at least two of the mesenteric vessels, since collateral circulation otherwise prevents the onset of symptoms; in more than 85% of cases, both the celiac artery and SMA are involved.[10]

Women are more commonly affected than men. Physical examination may reveal an epigastric bruit in about 50% of patients. Other atherosclerotic risk factors are often present. In addition, patients may demonstrate evidence of gallbladder dysmotility, gastroparesis, or gastric ulcers as a reflection of disease involving the celiac artery.[10, 14]

Venous Thrombosis

Venous thrombosis presentations vary from acute to chronic. The pain is more prominent in acute thrombosis, and bowel infarction is more likely in this group. Chronic thrombosis is usually painless and is associated with collaterals and varices.

Differential Diagnosis

The differential diagnosis in patients presenting with these symptoms is broad and includes some of the conditions described in Table 4.1. Table 4.2, on the other hand, provides clues to the differentiation between arterial and venous mesenteric thrombosis. Table 4.3 provides insight into different clinical features in acute mesenteric ischemia.

DIAGNOSTIC EVALUATION

Laboratory Data

Laboratory test results are nonspecific, especially early in the course. Common findings can include leukocytosis, acidemia with elevated anion gap, and elevated hematocrit resulting from hemoconcentration. Interest has been placed on elevated lactate levels, a reflection of ongoing anaerobic metabolism, suggestive of an ischemic

Table 4.1   Differential Diagnosis of Diffuse Abdominal Pain

Mesenteric or splanchnic insufficiency or infarction

Mesenteric venous thrombosis

Aortic aneurysm

Pancreatitis

Intestinal obstruction

Diverticulitis

Gallbladder disease

Early appendicitis

Gastroenteritis

Peritonitis

Inflammatory bowel disease

Irritable bowel

Mesenteric adenitis

Sickle cell crisis

Trauma

Pneumonia

Urinary tract infection

Pelvic inflammatory disease

Acute intermittent porphyria

Tabes dorsalis

Vasculitis (polyaarteritis nodosa, Henoch-Schönlein purpura)

Adrenal insufficiency

Metabolic (toxins, lead poisoning, uremia, drug overdose, diabetic ketoacidosis, heavy metal poisoning)

Table 4.2   Comparison of Acute Mesenteric Venous Thrombosis and Acute Mesenteric Arterial Thromboembolism

Variable	Venous Thrombosis	Arterial Thromboembolism
Risk factors	Prothrombotic states	Atherosclerotic vascular disease
	Inflammatory bowel disease	Valvular heart disease
	Abdominal cancer	Arrhythmias
Abdominal pain	Insidious onset	Sudden onset with embolic disease
Tests		
• Plain films	Usually non-specific	Usually non-specific
• Computed tomography	Sensitivity of more than 90%	Sensitivity of approximately 60%
• Mesenteric angiography	Not usually required for diagnosis	Often helpful
Involvement of inferior mesenteric vessels	Uncommon	Common

Operative findings		
• Mesenteric arterial pulsations	Preserved except late in disease	Absent
• Type of transition from ischemic to normal bowel	Gradual	Abrupt
Therapy		
• Thrombolysis	Rarely useful	Often useful
• Long-term anticoagulation	Indicated	Indicated
Sequelae	Short bowel, varices	Short bowel

Table adapted from reference 5.

Table 4.3 Clinical Features of Acute Mesenteric Ischemia

CAUSE	INCIDENCE (%)	PRESENTATION	RISK FACTORS	TREATMENT
Arterial embolism	40–50	Acute catastrophe	Arrhythmia, myocardial infarction, rheumatic valve disease, endocarditis, cardiomyopathies, ventricular aneurysms, history of embolic events, recent angiography	Embolectomy, papaverine, excise infarction
Arterial thrombosis	25	Insidious onset with progression to constant pain	Atherosclerosis, prolonged hypotension, estrogen, hypercoagulability	Papaverine, thrombectomy, excise infarction, revascularization
Non-occlusive	20	Acute or subacute	Hypovolemia, hypotension, low cardiac output state, alpha-adrenergic agonists, digoxin, beta-receptor blocking agents	Treat cause first, papaverine, excise dead bowel
Venous thrombosis	10	Subacute	Right-sided heart failure, previous deep vein thrombosis, hepatosplenomegaly, primary clotting disorder, malignancy, hepatitis, pancreatitis, recent abdominal surgery or infection, estrogen, polycythemia, sickle cell disease	Thrombectomy, excise dead bowel, heparinize, long-term complication

Table adapted from reference 12.

process. However, it is not specific for mesenteric ischemia.[12] Amylase is elevated in approximately 50% of patients. Fecal occult blood in the stool is present in 25% of patients.[2]

Hypercoagulability workup may help guide long-term therapy but is not helpful in the acute setting.

Recently, plasma D-dimer has been suggested as an early marker of acute ischemia based on animal studies. Similarly, the enzyme alcohol dehydrogenase has been identified as a potentially sensitive indicator of bowel ischemia.[9]

Imaging

Useful information can be gathered from imaging techniques. These studies may be indicated for the general evaluation of abdominal pain or for the specific evaluation of suspected mesenteric and splanchnic artery disease. However, if bowel infarction is suspected, urgent surgical therapy is mandated and should not be delayed to obtain imaging studies.

Plain radiographs are normal in a large proportion of patients. Findings suggestive of bowel ischemia/necrosis include ileus, bowel-wall thickening, or intramural gas. Intraluminal barium should not be used because it is rarely helpful in making a positive diagnosis and will interfere with angiographic studies.

Ultrasound

Transabdominal ultrasound can identify the mesenteric vessels and characterize its flow by using Doppler techniques (Figure 4.4).

Established criteria for the diagnosis of mesenteric stenosis focus on the peak systolic velocity (PSV) and end diastolic velocity (EDV) as measured by duplex ultrasonography. An EDV greater than 45 cm/s is 100% sensitive for the detection of stenosis > 50% in the superior mesenteric artery. Celiac artery stenosis can be detected indirectly in conjunction with the presence of reversal of the hepatic vein waveform, with retrograde common hepatic flow being the most sensitive indicator. Other studies argue that the PSV offers greater sensitivity than EDV in diagnosing stenosis of the SMA or celiac artery, with respective velocities greater than 275 cm/s and 200 cm/s indicating greater than 70% stenosis in these vessels.[15]

Ultrasound has several disadvantages. First, the inferior mesenteric artery is often difficult to visualize with duplex ultrasonography; nonetheless, mesenteric ischemia is rare in the presence of normal flow in the celiac and SMA.[14] Ultrasonography requires a skilled technologist and may be limited by patient body habitus, previous intra-abdominal surgeries, and the presence of bowel gas. Evaluation following a fasting period of 8 hours is often recommended for an optimal study, limiting its applicability in emergency situations. Therefore, ultrasound may be more suitable for evaluation of chronic mesenteric ischemia.[15]

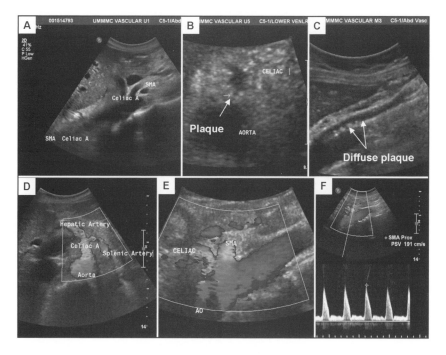

Figure 4.4

Duplex ultrasound of the celiac and mesenteric vessels. Panel A: Two-dimensional longitudinal view of the aorta at the origin of the celiac and superior mesenteric artery (SMA). Panel B: Transverse two-dimensional view of the aorta reveals calcified plaque at the origin of the celiac artery. Panel C: Longitudinal two-dimensional view of a superior mesenteric artery with diffuse calcified plaque. Panel D: Transverse two-dimensional and color Doppler view of the aorta at the level of the celiac artery and its bifurcation into the hepatic and splenic arteries. Panel E: Longitudinal two-dimensional and color Doppler view of the aorta at the level of the celiac and SMA origin. Panel F: Normal color and spectral Doppler profile in the superior mesenteric artery. **See Plate 5 for color image.**

Images courtesy of Denise Kush, RDMS, RVT; Vascular Laboratory, UMass Memorial Health Care.

Computed tomography

Early evaluations of mesenteric ischemia by CT showed a sensitivity of only 65%. Subsequently, the development of multidetector CT has greatly improved the sensitivity and specificity to nearly 95%.[16] In addition to findings of vessel occlusion or significant stenosis on CT angiography, associated changes in the bowel wall (i.e., wall thickening, mucosal enhancement, pneumatosis intestinalis, bowel loop dilatation) offer clues to the diagnosis (Figures 4.5 to 4.7).

Magnetic resonance imaging

MRI and MRA can be used to evaluate patients with acute mesenteric ischemia; however, it is time consuming, limiting its applicability in emergency situations. MRI is also

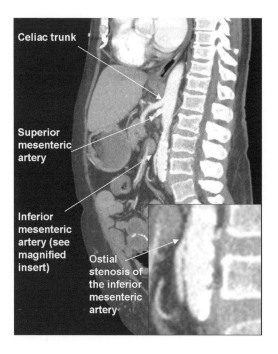

Figure 4.5

Sagittal CT angiography reveals an ostial stenosis of the inferior mesenteric artery.

useful in the evaluation of chronic mesenteric ischemia. MRI findings include abnormal postprandial blood flow and decreased bowel enhancement in bowel territories served by arteries with significant stenoses (Figure 4.8).[17, 18]

Angiography

Angiography is the gold standard for the diagnosis of mesenteric artery disease. It also offers the potential for therapeutic interventions for mesenteric ischemia. With strong clinical suspicion, workup should proceed directly to angiography, without delay for CT scan or other testing.

Typically, aortography is performed with anterior and lateral views. Lateral films provide optimal visualization for detecting proximal disease, permitting analysis of the takeoff of the celiac, the SMA, and the IMA (Figure 4.9).[10] Anterior views are helpful to diagnose ischemia caused by poor perfusion in the distal mesenteric vessels.[12]

When non-occlusive ischemia is suggested by angiography, intra-arterial infusion of vasodilators such as papaverine or prostaglandin E1 may also be used to augment blood flow if a test dose suggests the limitations in flow are reversible by augmenting arterial flow.[19]

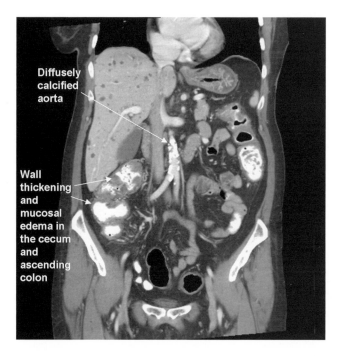

Diffusely calcified aorta

Wall thickening and mucosal edema in the cecum and ascending colon

Figure 4.6

Coronal CT of the abdomen reveals a calcified aorta and diffuse edema in the cecum and ascending colon with mucosal edema, findings which are suggestive of mesenteric ischemia.

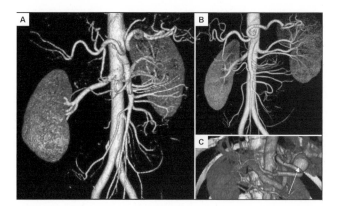

Figure 4.7

Three-dimensional computed tomography angiography of the abdominal vasculature. Panels A and B: Normal three-dimensional reconstructions in right anterior oblique and antero-posterior views, respectively. Panel C: Three-dimensional reconstruction of a splenic artery aneurysm (arrow).

Figures courtesy of David J. Sheehan, DO; Radiology Department, University of Massachusetts Medical Center and Medical School.

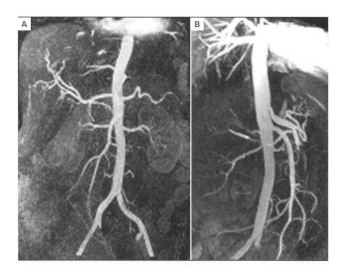

Figure 4.8

Magnetic Resonance Angiography of the mesenteric vessels. Panel A: Coronal two-dimensional view. Panel B: Sagittal two-dimensional view.

Figures courtesy of Raul Galvez, MD, MPH and Hale Ersoy, MD; Radiology Department, Brigham and Women's Hospital, Harvard Medical School.

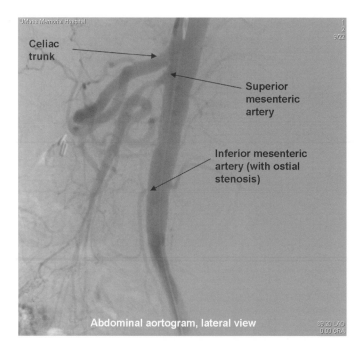

Figure 4.9

Digital substraction angiography in a patient with an ostial stenosis of the inferior mesenteric artery.

Mesenteric venous thrombosis may be suggested by a slowing in arterial inflow and filling defects in mesenteric veins or absent flow in veins with collateral routes of drainage.[19]

Finally, angiography may be the best diagnostic modality to confirm the diagnosis of median arcuate ligament syndrome, in which dynamic compression of the celiac artery is demonstrated with a combination of inspiratory and expiratory images.[11]

THERAPEUTIC CONSIDERATIONS

Medical Treatment of Mesenteric Artery Disease

The initial management should include hemodynamic monitoring and support, correction of acidemia, administration of broad-spectrum antibiotics, and gastric decompression via a nasogastric tube. Patients who have suspected mesenteric ischemia should receive adequate fluid resuscitation, because capillary leak in the setting of visceral ischemia may lead to significant fluid shifts. Vasoconstricting agents should be avoided to prevent exacerbating visceral ischemia. When vasopressors are required, preference should be given to beta-adrenergic agonists such as dopamine. Empiric, broad-spectrum antibiotics (e.g., imipenem) are recommended, because ischemia leads to more frequent translocation of bacteria through the intestinal wall.[8, 12]

Systemic anticoagulation remains the mainstay of non-operative therapy, and early use of heparin has been associated with improved survival.[5] Heparin is commonly reinstituted postoperatively when safe; long-term anticoagulation is strongly recommended for those who have ischemia caused by embolic events or mesenteric venous thrombosis to prevent reoccurrence.[8]

The ultimate goal of treatment is to restore blood flow to ischemic bowel as soon as possible, prior to the occurrence of infarction.

In the presence of signs of peritonitis, urgent laparotomy with resection of infarcted bowel is indicated.

When an SMA embolus is the culprit, embolectomy is considered standard treatment, in the absence of peritoneal signs. Depending on the location and degree of occlusion of the embolus, surgical revascularization, intra-arterial infusion of thrombolytic or vasodilator agents (e.g., tolazoline or papaverine), or systemic anticoagulation may be considered.[12]

In cases of in-situ SMA thrombosis, emergency surgical revascularization is the treatment of choice.

In patients with mesenteric vein thrombosis, treatment is dependent on the presence or absence of peritoneal signs. Laparotomy and resection of infarcted bowel in more advanced cases or, if there are no peritoneal signs, immediate anticoagulant therapy with heparin may be adequate.

The use of aspirin, thienopyridines, statins, or other cardiovascular medications have not been evaluated in patients with mesenteric ischemia, either acute or chronic. However, this population commonly has other cardiovascular comorbidities and indications for these medications.

Interventional Treatment

There are no randomized or controlled trials of diagnosis or therapy for intestinal ischemia, acute or chronic, regardless of cause.[2]

Percutaneous management of mesenteric ischemia

Few studies have compared percutaneous transluminal angioplasty (PTA) with surgery for mesenteric ischemia.

In one study of 28 patients undergoing percutaneous intervention compared with a total of 85 patients treated with various surgical procedures (mesenteric artery bypass, endarterectomy, or patch angioplasty), the morbidity and mortality between the two groups did not differ, although recurrence of symptoms was higher in the group treated percutaneously.[20]

In a second, smaller study, nine patients who underwent mesenteric bypass grafting were compared with eight patients who underwent angioplasty alone. There was no difference in mortality. Technical success, however, was achieved in only 30% of the PTA patients. Long-term pain relief occurred in 88% of the operative bypass group at 34.5 months, as compared with 67% in the angioplasty group at just 9 months (Table 4.4).[21]

Although one study documenting outcome following percutaneous transluminal angioplasty (PTA) of mesenteric vessels versus PTA with stenting found no difference in outcome, the overall trend has been toward increased use of PTA with stenting.[22] Table 4.5 summarizes findings of various PTA trials.

Thrombolytic therapy has been used as an adjunct to endovascular techniques (Figure 4.10). As with other endovascular techniques, peritoneal findings suggestive of bowel infarction remain a contraindication to thrombolysis and require surgical exploration. However, the data are mostly from case reports and small series with fewer than 50 patients reported in the literature.[3]

In patients with non-occlusive ischemia, the supraselective administration of papaverine (30 to 60 cc/hr) has resulted in a 20% reduction in mortality. Iloprost is being investigated in this population.[9]

Figure 4.11 offers a suggested algorithm for the management of acute mesenteric ischemia.

In patients undergoing angioplasty with stenting, dual-antiplatelet therapy is usually recommended for a period of 4 weeks.[23]

Table 4.4 Single-Institution Comparisons of Mesenteric Angioplasty/Stenting Versus Surgery

Author and Procedure	Year	N	Successfully Revascularized (%)	30-day Mortality (%)	Mean Follow-up	Recurrence (%)
Kasirajan	2001					
Angioplasty		28	93	11	3 yrs.	27
Surgery (historic controls)		85	98	8	3 yrs.	24
Rose	1995					
Angioplasty/ stenting		8	80	13	9 mos.	33
Surgery		9	100	11	3 yrs.	22
Bowser	2002					
Angioplasty/ stenting		18	88	11	14 mos.	46
Surgery		22	100	9	14 mos.	19

Table adapted from reference 2.

Table 4.5 Outcomes of Selected Series of Endovascular Treatment for Chronic Mesenteric Ischemia

Author	Year	N	Technical Success (%)	Clinical Success (%)	Procedural Complications (%)	Mortality (%)	Patency at Mean Follow-up (%)	Follow-up (mos.)
Kasirajan	2001	28	85.7	66	0	1	73	15
Matsumoto	2002	33	81.3	82	13	0	83.3	38
Shih	2003	33	87	88	13	3.4	83	11
Sharafuddin	2003	25	96	88	12	4	83	15
AbuRahama	2003	24	96	95	0	0	61	26
Landis	2005	29	97	90	13.7	6	70.1	12
Silva	2006	61	96	88	3.4	1.7	71	14
Atkins	2007	31	N/A	88	0	1	58	36

N/A = not available. Table adapted with data from references 2, 23, and 24.

Surgical therapy

Bypass may be antegrade, with inflow from the supraceliac aorta, or retrograde from the iliac vessels. Some investigators suggest that the former is more anatomically favorable, because retrograde grafts may be more prone to kinking. At exploration, unless bowel is necrotic, revascularization should be performed before bowel resection. Once revascularized, the bowel can be re-examined to determine if restoration of blood flow has reversed the ischemic process.

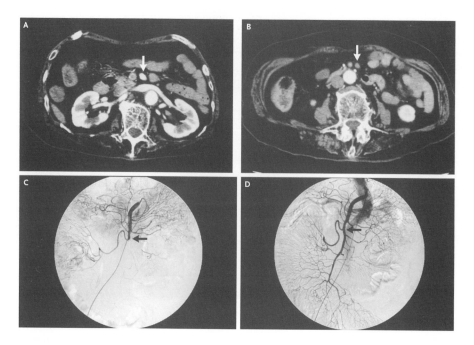

Figure 4.10

Computed tomographies (Panels A and B) and angiographies (panels C and D) in a patient with an occluded superior mesenteric artery treated with intra-arterial thrombolytics. Panels A and B reveal occlusion of the superior mesenteric artery. Abdominal angiography showed complete occlusion of the superior mesenteric artery (Panel C, arrow). Panel D reveals recanalization of the superior mesenteric artery after intra-arterial injection of urokinase and transcatheter thrombus aspiration.

Although reversed saphenous vein grafts are more appropriate in the setting of gross contamination from infarcted bowel,[25] prosthetic grafts may in fact be more durable for mesenteric artery bypass. No randomized trials exist regarding the use of prosthetic versus endogenous grafts, but most series indicate a preference for the use of prosthetic grafts. Synthetic grafts also offer the benefit of facilitating simultaneous revascularization of the celiac and SMA through a single aortotomy with the use of bifurcated grafts. Although not proven by randomized studies, revascularization of both vessels appears to provide redundancy and better outcomes. Embolectomy can also be performed during surgery.

Patency results of mesenteric bypass graft are favorable, with 89%–94% 5-year patency rates in two small series.[26, 27] Symptom-free survival rates range from 57% to 86% at 5 years.

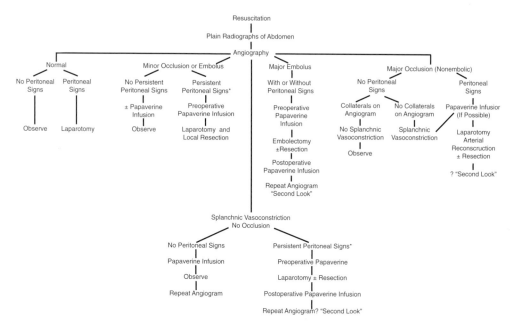

Figure 4.11

Suggested algorithm for the diagnosis and treatment of patients at risk of acute mesenteric ischemia. Emergency laparotomy may be justified without angiography when the clinical suggestion of bowel ischemia is high. Asterisk indicates that peritoneal signs are considered persistent if they are not relieved within 30 minutes of receiving a dose of tolazoline.

Determination of bowel viability is critical in surgical therapy for mesenteric ischemia. Clinical assessment of bowel color and motility remains the best method. Other techniques, including antimesenteric Doppler interrogation, and observation of perfusion following administration of intravenous fluorescein dye, are commonly used. None of these, however, predict future intestinal viability, and they have a sensitivity of less than 60%.[28] Because of the inability to predict which segments of bowel remain viable, a second-look operation 24 to 48 hours after the initial procedure has been historically recommended.[28]

Surgery is the preferred method for patients with median arcuate ligament syndrome. It consists of release of the ligament, with or without placement of a bypass. Endovascular therapies have failed because stents are usually compressed by the ligament.[22]

◇◇◇◇◇◇◇◇◇◇◇◇

REFERENCES

1. Rosenblum JD, Boyle CM, Schwartz LB. The mesenteric circulation: anatomy and physiology. *Surg Clin North Am.* 1997;77:289–306.

2. Hirsch AT, Haskal ZJ, Hertzer NR, et al. ACC/AHA 2005 Practice Guidelines for the management of patients with peripheral arterial disease (lower extremity, renal, mesenteric, and abdominal aortic): a collaborative report from the American Association for Vascular Surgery/Society for Vascular Surgery, Society for Cardiovascular Angiography and Interventions, Society for Vascular Medicine and Biology, Society of Interventional Radiology, and the ACC/AHA Task Force on Practice Guidelines (Writing Committee to Develop Guidelines for the Management of Patients with Peripheral Arterial Disease): Endorsed by the American Association of Cardiovascular and Pulmonary Rehabilitation; National Heart, Lung, and Blood Institute; Society for Vascular Nursing; TransAtlantic Inter-Society Consensus; and Vascular Disease Foundation. *Circulation.* 2006;113:e463–e654.

3. Schoots IG, Levi MM, Reekers JA, Lameris JS, van Gulik TM. Thrombolytic therapy for acute superior mesenteric artery occlusion. *J Vasc Interv Radiol.* 2005;16:317–329.

4. Schoots IG, Koffeman GI, Legemate DA, Levi M, van Gulik TM. Systematic review of survival after acute mesenteric ischaemia according to disease aetiology. *Br J Surg.* 2004;91:17–27.

5. Kumar S, Sarr MG, Kamath PS. Mesenteric venous thrombosis. *N Engl J Med.* 2001;345:1683–1688.

6. Mamode N, Pickford I, Leiberman P. Failure to improve outcome in acute mesenteric ischaemia: seven-year review. *Eur J Surg.* 1999;165:203–208.

7. Acosta S, Ogren M, Sternby NH, Bergqvist D, Bjorck M. Incidence of acute thrombo-embolic occlusion of the superior mesenteric artery—a population-based study. *Eur J Vasc Endovasc Surg.* 2004;27:145–150.

8. Falkensammer J, Oldenburg WA. Surgical and medical management of mesenteric ischemia. *Curr Treat Options Cardiovasc Med.* 2006;8:137–143.

9. Chang RW, Chang JB, Longo WE. Update in management of mesenteric ischemia. *World J Gastroenterol.* 2006;12:3243–3247.

10. Moawad J, Gewertz BL. Chronic mesenteric ischemia: clinical presentation and diagnosis. *Surg Clin North Am.* 1997;77:357–369.

11. Sharafuddin MJ, Olson CH, Sun S, Kresowik TF, Corson JD. Endovascular treatment of celiac and mesenteric arteries stenoses: applications and results. *J Vasc Surg.* 2003;38:692–698.

12. Oldenburg WA, Lau LL, Rodenberg TJ, Edmonds HJ, Burger CD. Acute mesenteric ischemia: a clinical review. *Arch Intern Med.* 2004;164:1054–1062.

13. Ottinger LW. The surgical management of acute occlusion of the superior mesenteric artery. *Ann Surg.* 1978;188:721–731.

14. Kazmers A. Operative management of chronic mesenteric ischemia. *Ann Vasc Surg.* 1998;12:299–308.

15. Nicoloff AD, Williamson WK, Moneta GL, Taylor LM, Porter JM. Duplex ultrasonography in evaluation of splanchnic artery stenosis. *Surg Clin North Am.* 1997;77:339–355.

16. Levy AD. Mesenteric ischemia. *Radiologic Clin North Am.* 2007;45:593.

17. Li KC. Chronic mesenteric ischemia: evaluation with phase-contrast cine MR imaging. *Radiology.* 1994; 190:175.

18. Lauenstein TC. MR imaging of apparent small-bowel perfusion for diagnosing mesenteric ischemia: feasibility study. *Radiology.* 2005;234:569.

19. Clark RA, Gallant TE. Acute mesenteric ischemia: Angiographic spectrum. *AJR Am J Roentgenol.* 1984;142: 555–562.

20. Kasirajan K. Chronic mesenteric ischemia: open surgery versus percutaneous angioplasty and stenting. *J Vasc Surg.* 2001;33:63.

21. Rose SC. Revascularization for chronic mesenteric ischemia: comparison of operative arterial bypass grafting and percutaneous transluminal angioplasty. *J Vasc Interven Rad.* 1995;6:339.

22. Shih MC, Angle JF, Leung DA, et al. CTA and MRA in mesenteric ischemia: Part 2, normal findings and complications after surgical and endovascular treatment. *AJR Am J Roentgenol.* 2007;188: 462–471.

23. Kougias P, El Sayed HF, Zhou W, Lin PH. Management of chronic mesenteric ischemia: the role of endovascular therapy. *J Endovasc Ther.* 2007;14: 395–405.

24. Schreiber T, Gardi D, Penugonda N. Percutaneous intervention of superior mesenteric artery stenosis in elderly patients. *Clin Cardiol.* 2009;32:232.

25. Shanley CJ, Ozaki CK, Zelenock GB. Bypass grafting for chronic mesenteric ischemia. *Surg Clin North Am.* 1997;77:381–395.

26. Jimenez JG, Huber TS, Ozaki CK, et al. Durability of antegrade synthetic aortomesenteric bypass for chronic mesenteric ischemia. *J Vasc Surg.* 2002;35: 1078–1084.

27. McMillan WD, McCarthy WJ, Bresticker MR, et al. Mesenteric artery bypass: objective patency determination. *J Vasc Surg.* 1995;21:729–740.

28. Ballard JL, Stone WM, Hallett JW, Pairolero PC, Cherry KJ. A critical analysis of adjuvant techniques used to assess bowel viability in acute mesenteric ischemia. *Am Surg.* 1993;59:309–311.

CHAPTER 5
Subclavian Artery Disease

UPPER EXTREMITY VASCULAR ANATOMY

Subclavian Artery

The subclavian arteries supply arterial flow to the upper extremities. Typically, the left subclavian artery arises directly from the aortic arch as the third and final of the great vessels, while the right subclavian artery arises from the bifurcation of the innominate artery (Figure 5.1). The innominate and left subclavian arteries typically arise from the horizontal portion of the arch, although there is considerable individual difference in the location of, and distance between, the origins of the great vessels (see types of aortic arch in Chapter 6).

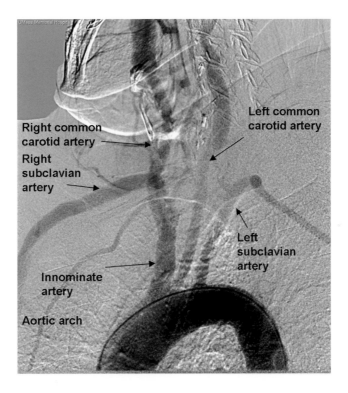

Figure 5.1

Digital substraction angiography reveals the anatomy of the aortic arch branch vessels.

The subclavian artery extends from its origin to the lateral border of the first rib. Traditionally, the artery is divided into three segments based on their relationship to the scalenus anterior muscle. The most important branches arise from the first segment and include the vertebral artery, internal thoracic artery, and thyrocervical trunk. The vertebral and internal thoracic arteries are largely constant between individuals in their origin and course, arising as the first and second branches, respectively. Typically, the right and left vertebral arteries are asymmetric in size, with a dominant vessel contributing most of the flow to the basilar artery. In contrast, the thyrocervical trunk varies widely between individuals in terms of the pattern and size of its branches.

The origination of the right subclavian artery as the terminal arch vessel from the descending thoracic aorta is seen in 0.5% of people. A bovine origin of the left common carotid artery off the innominate artery occurs in approximately 7%–20% of people and is relevant in angiography of the right subclavian artery. The most common anomaly of subclavian artery branches is origination of the left vertebral artery directly from the aortic arch (0.5%–6%).

Axillary Artery

The axillary artery is a direct continuation of the subclavian artery. It extends from the lateral border of the first rib to the inferior border of the teres major muscle. The bony landmark for this inferior margin is the anatomical neck of the humerus. The branches of the axillary artery demonstrate significant interindividual variation (Figure 5.2).

Brachial Artery

The brachial artery is the direct continuation of the axillary artery. It extends from the inferior border of the teres major muscle (anatomical neck of the humerus) to the neck of the radius. The profunda brachii branch of the brachial artery descends posteriorly in the arm and contributes to the elbow collateral circulation. The other major branches of the brachial artery include muscular branches to the arm muscles, the nutrient artery to the humerus, and collateral vessels to the elbow (Figure 5.2).

Ulnar Artery

The ulnar artery is the major vessel to the forearm and is usually larger than the radial artery. It arises from the brachial artery bifurcation and extends from the neck of the radius to the pisiform carpal bone. Its main branch is the interosseous, which supplies the interosseous membrane and forearm muscles. In addition, the ulnar artery supplies collateral branches to the elbow, muscular branches to the forearm, and carpal branches to the palmar and dorsal aspect of the wrist; contributes to the deep palmar arch; and continues into the hand as the major source of blood flow to the superficial palmar arch (Figures 5.3 and 5.4).

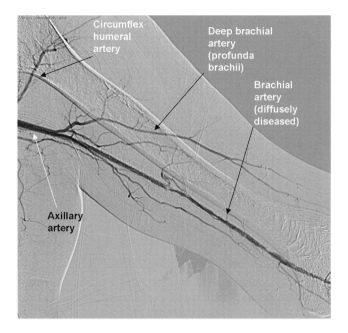

Figure 5.2

Digital substraction angiography revealing the arterial tree of the arm.

Radial Artery

The radial artery is the smaller of the terminal branches of the brachial artery. It extends from the neck of the radius to the styloid process of the radius. Like the ulnar artery, the radial artery contributes collaterals to the elbow, muscular branches to the forearm, and carpal branches to the palmar and dorsal aspects of the wrist. In the hand, it contributes to the superficial palmar arch and continues into the hand as the major source of blood flow to the deep palmar arch (Figures 5.3 and 5.4).

Arterial Supply to the Hand

The arterial supply of the hand is provided by the superficial and deep palmar arches. The deep arch is primarily formed from the terminal portion of the radial artery and is complete in 95% of individuals. The superficial arch is primarily formed from the terminal portion of the ulnar artery and is complete in 80% of patients. Angiographically, the deep arch lies proximal to the superficial arch and is generally less prominent. Common palmar digital arteries arise from the superficial arch and fuse with palmar metacarpal branches from the deep arch. In the interdigital space, each of the common palmar digital arteries then

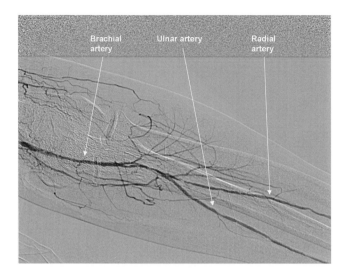

Figure 5.3

Digital substraction angiography of the brachial bifurcation into the ulnar and radial arteries.

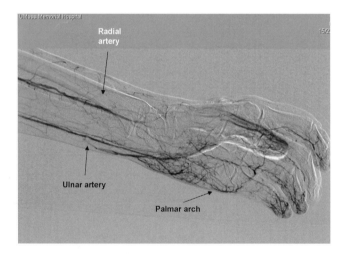

Figure 5.4

Digital substraction angiography of the forearm arterial tree.

divides into two proper palmar digital arteries, which run along the sides of the second to fifth digits and supply the arterial network of the finger pads. The thumb usually receives a direct branch from the terminal portion of the radial artery (Figure 5.4).[1]

ETIOLOGY AND PATHOPHYSIOLOGY

Most cases of subclavian artery disease (SAD) are due to atherosclerotic disease. Etiologies, such as inflammatory diseases and traumatic or congenital causes of sub-clavian stenosis, appear to be responsible for fewer than 5% of cases. Fibromuscular dysplasia affecting the subclavian artery is also unusual.[2, 3] (See Chapters 1 and 2). Table 5.1 summarizes the different etiologies of SAD.

Vascular Thoracic Outlet Syndrome

Thoracic outlet syndrome (TOS) refers to compression of the neurovascular structures of the arm (brachial plexus, subclavian artery, and vein) as they leave the thoracic outlet. A high incidence (> 50%) of cervical ribs or anomalous ligamentous bands has been reported in patients with subclavian arterial compression. While vascular complications of this syndrome are uncommon, occurring in < 10% of patients with TOS, they account for most of the serious morbidity associated with this condition. Trauma to the artery can lead to progressive stenosis and occlusion.

EPIDEMIOLOGY/NATURAL HISTORY

Prevalence and Risk Factors

In contrast to peripheral, renal, or carotid artery disease, there are no large epidemiologic studies of SAD. It is a condition that may be under-recognized because of its atypical clinical presentation.

Brachiocephalic or subclavian artery obstructions are thought to account for up to 17% of symptomatic extracranial cerebrovascular disease.[10]

Table 5.1 Causes of Subclavian Artery Disease

Atherosclerosis
Congenital abnormalities
Vasculitis
Thoracic outlet syndrome
Radiation-induced stenosis
Aneurysmal disease
Fibromuscular dysplasia
Post-surgical or post-trauma complications
Acute intimal dissection (spontaneous, traumatic, or iatrogenic)

Adapted from references 4–9.

In a retrospective study of 23,500 patients, the incidence of subclavian stenosis or occlusion in patients examined in a vascular laboratory was 1.15%.[3]

A large epidemiologic study of SAD pooled analyses of four different cohorts. In this study of 4,223 patients, in which subclavian artery stenosis (SAS) was defined as a > 15 mmHg of interarm blood pressure difference, the prevalence of SAS was 1.9% in two general population cohorts, and 7.1% in two cohorts consisting of patients being evaluated in non-invasive vascular laboratories for any reason. Subclavian stenosis was associated with previous or current smoking, hypertension, lower HDL cholesterol levels, or the presence of peripheral artery disease (Table 5.2).[11]

The incidence of SAD increases in patients with other cardiovascular comorbidities. Among patients with peripheral vascular disease, a small angiographic series of 48 patients demonstrated that 19% had significant (> 50%) stenosis of the subclavian artery.[12] SAD also appears to be more frequent in patients with more advanced coronary artery disease.

There appears to be a preponderance of left subclavian involvement over the right subclavian or the innominate artery, yet up to a third of stenoses may involve right innominate or subclavian arteries.[3, 11]

CABG Population

The reported incidence of SAD in patients for whom coronary artery bypass graft surgery (CABG) is contemplated with the use of an internal mammary graft to the left anterior descending artery varies depending upon the population studied. In unselected populations, the incidence ranges from 0.5% to 6.8%.[13–16] Patients with clinical evidence of peripheral arterial disease (PAD) have significantly higher rates of SAD, ranging from 11.8% to 18.7%.[17] The incidence of coronary subclavian steal syndrome (defined as angiographic evidence of retrograde internal mammary artery flow) after CABG has been reported as high as 3.4%.[18]

Table 5.2   Risk Factors for Atherosclerotic Subclavian Artery Disease

Risk Factor	Odds Ratio
Cigarette use	
Former	1.80
Current	2.61
Hypertension	1.90 per 20 mmHg increase
Low HDL cholesterol	0.87 per 10 mg/dl decrease
Concomitant peripheral artery disease	5.11

Adapted with information from reference 11.

Clinical Outcomes in Patients with SAD

Subclavian artery disease is associated with increased mortality in all age groups. Mortality appears to increase with the degree of severity of SAD (Figures 5.5 to 5.8). Whether SAD is only a marker or an independent predictor of mortality remains to be determined.[19]

A pooled cohort study, consisting of two cohorts from non-invasive vascular laboratories and one from the general population, included 1800 patients who were followed for a mean of 10 years. Subclavian artery stenosis (SAS), defined as brachial systolic pressure difference $\geq$ 15 mmHg, was found in 8.8% of patients. The presence of SAS in multivariate analyses adjusting for multiple cardiovascular risk factors and treatments was

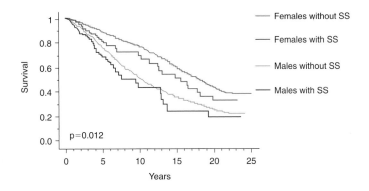

Figure 5.5

Twenty-five year survival according to gender and presence of subclavian stenosis (SS).

Reprinted from: J Am Coll Cardiol, Vol. 49, Aboyans V, Criqui MH, McDermott MM, et al., Pages 1540–5. Copyright, 2007, with permission from Elsevier.

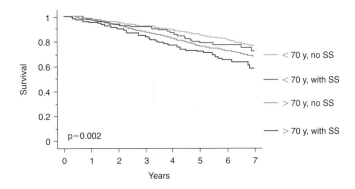

Figure 5.6

Seven-year survival according to age group and presence of subclavian stenosis.

Reprinted from: J Am Coll Cardiol, Vol. 49, Aboyans V, Criqui MH, McDermott MM, et al., Pages 1540–5. Copyright, 2007, with permission from Elsevier.

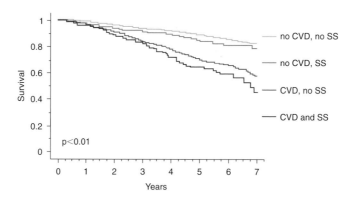

Figure 5.7

Seven-year survival according to presence of any cardiovascular disease (clinical and/or ABI < 0.9).

Reprinted from: J Am Coll Cardiol, Vol. 49, Aboyans V, Criqui MH, McDermott MM, et al., Pages 1540–5. Copyright, 2007, with permission from Elsevier.

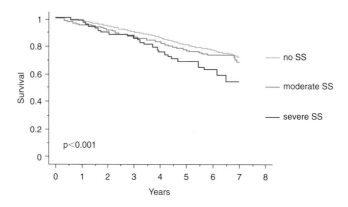

Figure 5.8

Seven-year survival according to subclavian stenosis severity.

Reprinted from: J Am Coll Cardiol, Vol. 49, Aboyans V, Criqui MH, McDermott MM, et al., Pages 1540–5. Copyright, 2007, with permission from Elsevier.

associated with increased total and cardiovascular disease mortality (hazard ratios 1.42 and 1.5, respectively). When any history of cardiovascular disease or PVD (defined as an ABI < 0.9) was added to the model, SAS remained an independent predictor of total mortality (hazard ratio 1.34) and had a non-significant trend towards increased cardiovascular mortality (hazard ratio 1.43).[19]

Patients with SAD and subclavian steal syndrome appear to have an increased risk of carotid artery disease and stroke. In a series of 55 patients with subclavian steal syndrome, followed for a mean of 4 years, 71% of patients had carotid artery disease progression, and 12% experienced either a stroke or a TIA during the follow-up period. Carotid endarterectomy was required in 10% of patients. In this series, no patient with SAD had a vertebrobasilar stroke, although 5% had vertebrobasilar TIAs.[20] This appears consistent with the findings of another retrospective study.[3]

Among patients with non-atherosclerotic SAD, the risk of stroke appears to be increased. In patients with Takayasu's arteritis, which involves the subclavian artery in most patients, a series of 88 patients followed for 6 years revealed that eight patients had stroke, two of whom died.[21] In this series it is not clear if the strokes were due to disease in other vascular territories or secondary to subclavian artery involvement.[22]

CLINICAL PRESENTATION

Claudication is defined as fatigue, discomfort, or pain that occurs in specific limb muscle groups during effort due to exercise-induced ischemia.[23] Arm claudication is frequently encountered in patients with SAD.

Patients with SAD may present with neurologic symptoms. In a study of 23,500 patients evaluated by continuous-wave Doppler ultrasound, 272 (1.15%) were found to have subclavian stenosis or occlusion. Of these, 54% were asymptomatic and had a normal neurological examination; 29% reported vertebrobasilar transient ischemic attacks (TIAs), with or without concomitant TIAs or infarction in the vascular territory of the carotid arteries; and 17% complained of symptoms exclusively referring to the region of carotid blood supply. Reversal of blood flow in the ipsilateral vertebral artery was detected in 152 patients (56%). The incidence of neurological symptoms within this group was double that found in patients without vertebrobasilar steal. Of note, none of the patients suffered from permanent vertebrobasilar damage in this study.[3]

Table 5.3 provides clues into the differential diagnosis and clinical presentation of SAD.

Thoracic Outlet Syndrome

The most typical clinical presentation of these patients is thromboembolism to the forearm and digits. Because of collateral formation, ischemic symptoms may be mild or absent.[1] Figure 5.9 outlines potential signs and symptoms of TOS.

Even in patients with vertebrobasilar symptoms or with evidence of vertebrobasilar retrograde flow, some suggest these symptoms have to be persistent or severe to warrant intervention, because as many as 50% of patients may have spontaneous remission of their symptoms.[24]

DIAGNOSTIC EVALUATION

Significant SAD is defined as a > 50% diameter stenosis in the subclavian artery.

Physical Exam

Current hypertension guidelines recommend an appropriate measurement of blood pressure with verification in the contralateral arm.[25] This may identify not only patients with pathology in the thoracic aorta, but also those with SAD.

Table 5.3   Differential Diagnosis and Clinical Presentation of Subclavian Artery Disease

Atherosclerosis
- Presentation as arm claudication
- Presentation as subclavian steal syndrome
  - Vertebrobasilar insufficiency
  - Chest pain in patients with internal mammary grafts
  - Lower extremity claudication in patients with axillofemoral bypass

Congenital abnormalities
- Vascular rings
- Aberrant origin of subclavian arteries

Vasculitis
- Takayasu's arteritis
- Giant cell arteritis
- Buerger's disease (thromboangiitis obliterans)

Thoracic outlet syndrome
- Arterial compression by cervical or first rib
- Macromastia

Radiation-induced stenosis

Subclavian aneurysm (due to cystic media necrosis)

Marfan's syndrome causing subclavian aneurysms

Sequelae of trauma (stenosis or aneurysm)

Infectious aneurysm (e.g., syphilis, tuberculosis)

Fibromuscular dysplasia

Paget-Schroetter syndrome (effort-related venous thrombosis)

Post-surgical complications (i.e., anastomotic-graft strictures)

Arteriovenous fistulas (traumatic or spontaneous)

Acute intimal dissection (spontaneous, traumatic, or iatrogenic)

Adapted from references 4–9.

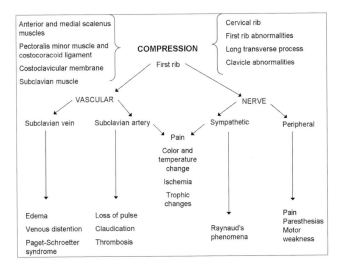

Figure 5.9

Compression factors in the thoracic outlet with potential signs and symptoms produced.

Reproduced from: Urschel HC Jr, Razzuk MA. Neurovascular compression in the thoracic outlet: changing management over 50 years. Ann Surg 1998;228:609–17 with permission from Wolters Kluwer Health/Lippincott, Williams & Wilkins.

Blood pressure measurements may be assisted with Doppler ultrasound. The use of an arm cuff and portable 5-MHz continuous-wave Doppler allows brachial pressures to be determined.

As a screening method, pressure difference between blood pressure readings in each upper extremity is not very sensitive, but it can be highly specific for SAD. In small case series inclusive of 17 patients with angiographically demonstrated SAD, a > 10 mmHg systolic blood pressure difference had a sensitivity of 65% and a specificity of 85%.[26] These were 35% and 94%, respectively, when a 20 mmHg gradient was used. Similarly, in a small series of 59 patients who were candidates for CABG, an upper extremity blood pressure difference of ≥ 15 mmHg identified all patients with ≥ 50% SAS.[27] Subsequent epidemiologic studies have used the 15 mmHg gradient definition.[19]

Duplex Ultrasound

The innominate and subclavian arteries are easily assessed by duplex scanning and pulsed-wave Doppler (Figure 5.10). It is important to be aware that the normal flow pattern in the upper extremity may be either biphasic or triphasic; this is unlike in the leg, where only a triphasic pattern is normal.[1, 28] Table 5.4 provides more details on the interpretation of subclavian and vertebral Duplex ultrasound.

Ultrasonography has the advantage of being relatively rapid and inexpensive, with no exposure to ionizing radiation. In addition, it can identify signs of early subclavian

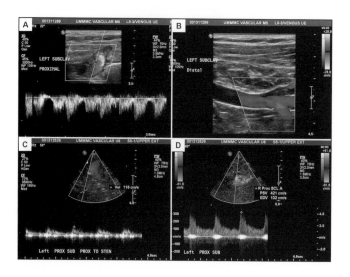

Figure 5.10

Subclavian arterial Duplex ultrasound. Panels A and B: Two-dimensional, spectral and color Doppler of a normal proximal and distal left subclavian artery. Panel C: Color and spectral Doppler of the left subclavian proximal to a stenotic segment reveal normal flow. Panel D: Color Doppler distal to a stenotic segment reveals aliasing, suggestive of turbulent flow; spectral Doppler indicates increased velocity of 4.2 meters per second, consistent with significant subclavian stenosis. **See Plate 6 for color image**.

Images courtesy of Denise Kush, RDMS, RVT; Vascular Laboratory, UMass Memorial Health Care.

Table 5.4   Interpretation of Subclavian and Vertebral Duplex Ultrasound

Subclavian artery	
Normal	Normal flow velocity Biphasic or triphasic waveform
< 50% stenosis	Flow velocity increased < 100 to 250 cm/s
50%–99% stenosis	Flow velocity increased > 100 to 250 cm/s, poststenotic color turbulence or aliasing
Occlusion	No flow detected
Vertebral artery	
< 50% stenosis	Normal flow velocity Biphasic or triphasic waveform
> 50% stenosis	Retrograde systolic flow Antegrade diastolic flow Low-amplitude velocity

Adapted from references 1 and 29.

steal, even in the absence of frank flow reversal.[30] For example, the presence of an early systolic deceleration or bidirectional flow can identify patients with latent subclavian steal.

The sensitivity of Duplex ultrasound of the subclavian artery and the vertebral artery to detect SAS > 50% is approximately 80%. Its negative predictive value is > 95%. In addition, duplex ultrasound is also highly useful in clinical follow-up of patients after revascularization.[29]

The major limitation of Doppler is its operator dependence.[30]

CT Angiography

Although there have been no direct comparisons of CT angiography versus conventional angiography specifically for subclavian stenosis, CT of the aortic arch and its branches appears to be highly sensitive and specific.[31] In addition, when the subclavian artery is not imaged in dedicated coronary CT angiography, the presence of poor left internal mammary artery (LIMA) opacification has been described as an indirect sign of subclavian steal.[32]

With regards to surveillance, multi-slice spiral CT angiography was found to have a sensitivity and specificity of 86% to identify restenosis in patients who underwent PTA with and without stenting when compared to a clinical questionnaire and blood pressure difference measurement.[33] No comparison to conventional angiography was made.

Major disadvantages of CT angiography are the use of potentially nephrotoxic contrast media and the exposure to ionizing radiation. Figure 5.11 provides an example of subclavian artery assessment by CT angiography.

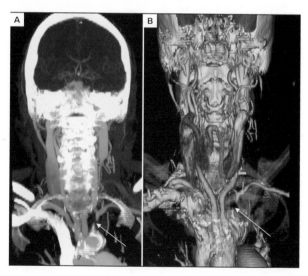

Figure 5.11

Computed tomography angiography in a patient with left subclavian artery occlusion and distal flow via the left vertebral artery. Panel A: Coronal two-dimensional maximum intensity projection. Panel B: Coronal three-dimensional reconstruction. Arrows indicate the site of occlusion.

Images courtesy of David J. Sheehan, DO; UMass Radiology Department.

Magnetic Resonance Angiography

Magnetic resonance angiography (MRA) has been useful in identifying patients with subclavian artery disease, particularly when patients present with neurovascular symptoms. It can also help differentiate other neurovascular pathologies (Figure 5.12).

In a small study comparing three-dimensional time-of-flight MRA with conventional angiography, MRA was found to have a sensitivity of 93% and a specificity of 89% for identifying > 50% stenoses.[34]

Time-of-flight MRA, however, is a time-consuming protocol and is inaccurate in states of slow flow. These difficulties can potentially be overcome with gadolinium-enhanced MRA, which can precisely image subclavian, carotid, and vertebral arteries without the problems of time-of-flight MRA.[35] Reported sensitivities and specificities for stenoses of more than 50% in the craniocervical vessels are close to 100% with the use of gadolinium. However, for imaging of the vertebral arteries, MRA has a sensitivity of only 85% when compared to angiography.[36]

MRA has the disadvantages of requiring long time consuming imaging sequences, being of a relatively high cost, and having limited access. Stents may cause significant artifact.

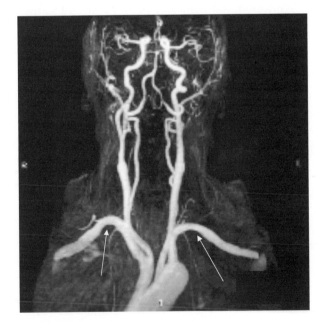

Figure 5.12

Magnetic Resonance Angiography of the subclavian arteries. Two dimensional view of the aortic arch and its branches. The innominate artery and the subclavian arteries (arrows) are easily visualized.

Figure courtesy of Raul Galvez, MD, MPH and Hale Ersoy, MD; Radiology Department, Brigham and Women's Hospital, Harvard Medical School.

When gadolinium is used, a potential risk of developing nephrogenic systemic fibrosis exists (further detailed in Chapter 2).

Even when cerebrovascular imaging is performed excluding the aortic arch and neck vessels, clinicians may use certain imaging findings to suspect subclavian or carotid disease. For example, the indirect finding of a hemispheric perfusion abnormality on MRI, with no corresponding intracranial stenosis on MRA of the circle of Willis, implies the presence of an upstream obstruction.[30]

Angiography

Angiography is the gold standard for the diagnosis of subclavian artery disease. The use of digital substraction is particularly useful to improve visualization of the arterial tree despite overlying bony structures. This technique has the disadvantage of being invasive, using ionizing radiation and potentially nephrotoxic contrast media. In addition, manipulation of the catheters in the aortic arch can be a cause of stroke.[1]

Thoracic outlet syndrome

Angiography is useful to confirm the site of the stenosis or occlusion and the presence of aneurysm formation, and to document the presence of distal embolization.[1]

Vasculitis

In patients with large-vessel vasculitis (e.g., temporal arteritis, Takayasu's arteritis), angiography is reserved for those with critical ischemia and is helpful to define the extent of disease involvement and the suitability for any revascularization procedure.

Angiography can also be useful for patients with small-vessel vasculitis in whom there is doubt regarding the diagnosis (e.g., a patient with atherosclerotic risk factors and asymmetric acronecrosis, in whom the absence of proximal lesions with thromboembolic potential and the presence of a symmetric bilateral process in the small vessels of the hand would be strong supportive evidence of vasculitis).

Apart from defining the vessel size affected, angiography is rarely helpful in differentiating between the various vasculitic processes.[1]

Patients Expected to Undergo Coronary Artery Bypass Graft Surgery

The prevalence of significant left SAD ranges from 0.5% to 6.8% at the time of cardiac catheterization, as described above.[16] This may have important implications at the time of CABG because of the potential risk of developing coronary steal syndrome.

Debate exists in the literature as to whether or not routine angiography of the left subclavian artery and/or left internal mammary artery (LIMA) should be performed in patients in whom CABG is contemplated. Arguments against routine angiography mention the fact that this procedure is not entirely benign. However, the complication rate is low, with the most common reported complications consisting of transient ischemic attacks or left upper extremity embolism in four large series with an incidence of 0% to 1.7%.[14–16, 37]

Alternatives to angiography include careful history taking and estimation of arm blood pressure differential. In a prospective study of 59 CABG candidates, bilateral arm blood pressure measurements, auscultation for supraclavicular or cervical bruits, and questioning about cerebrovascular symptoms were compared to brachiocephalic subclavian arteriography. Although all patients with significant stenosis were identified by a > 15 mmHg arm pressure difference, there were only four such patients in this study. One patient experienced a transient ischemic attack after subclavian angiography.[27]

Options for treatment include:

- Subclavian artery stenting.[16]
- Using a free LIMA graft, which in modern series has long-term (> 90%) patency rates comparable to an in-situ LIMA graft.[38]

THERAPEUTIC CONSIDERATIONS

Medical Treatment

Most of the patients with SAD have comorbidities such as diabetes, dyslipidemia, hypertension, coronary disease, or other peripheral vascular disease and should be aggressively treated, as described elsewhere in this book.

There have been no randomized trials evaluating treatment modalities for SAD (medical versus interventional, PTA with or without stenting versus surgery). All the treatment data described below are derived from prospective or retrospective series.

Only one retrospective study has evaluated outcomes of medical (not defined in the study) versus interventional treatment of SAD. In this study, 223 patients were followed for a median of 42 months. Patients treated with angioplasty had improved hemodynamic parameters of the stenotic vessel when evaluated by non-invasive studies on follow-up (Doppler and oscillography). However, the risk of having a symptomatic stenosis at the time of follow-up did not differ between the treatment groups.[39]

Although the use of aspirin, ticlopidine, and statins has been described in studies of SAD, there have been no meaningful outcome studies related to the use of these medications, and previous reports provide only anecdotal evidence.[40] The exception is one study from the surgical population: Aspirin appears to improve graft patency after carotid-subclavian bypass grafting, as evaluated retrospectively in 40 patients, who were followed for a mean of 61 months. Graft patency rates were 100% in patients receiving aspirin versus 60% in those not receiving antiplatelet agents.[41]

Interventional Treatment

The outcome of subclavian artery percutaneous revascularization has been exclusively reported from retrospective case series. No randomized studies have compared the outcome of percutaneous versus surgical revascularization, or the outcome for patients treated with angioplasty versus stenting. Table 5.5 summarizes current indications for revascularization in patients with SAD.

Percutaneous treatment of SAD

The evolution in technique and technology from angioplasty alone, to angioplasty with provisional stenting, and finally to angioplasty and stenting in all cases reflects the improved outcomes achieved with stenting. The technical success rate in contemporary series approaches 100%. The success rate for total occlusions has improved dramatically over the last decade and can approach 90%. Table 5.6 summarizes selected reported case series.

The risk of cerebral embolization or embolization to the ipsilateral limb or IMA artery has been consistently low (< 1%) or absent in all of these series. The rarity of embolism to the vertebral artery is probably explained by the delay in the re-establishment of antegrade flow following relief of the proximal obstruction (20 seconds to 20 minutes).[17] When cerebral events occur, they are more often related to manipulation of the aortic arch than to stenting of the subclavian artery itself. Limb embolization typically occurs in the digits.[1]

Access-site complications are the most common serious adverse events reported (0%–7%) and are closely related to the use of the brachial artery for access. Complications of percutaneous treatment include dissection, pseudo-aneurysm, distal embolization, and vessel rupture.[42, 43] Approximately half of these complications will require operative repair. Stent migration is an uncommon complication. Although not specifically reported in all of these series, stent migration may occur during deployment, particularly of self-expanding stents. This may result in covering ("jailing") of the vertebral artery ostium. The consequence of this will depend on whether there is resultant plaque

Table 5.5   Indications for Subclavian Artery Revascularization

Upper extremity symptoms
- Incapacitating arm claudication
- Upper limb ischemia
- Distal embolization

Subclavian steal syndrome
- Coronary: angina despite adequate medical therapy; moderate to large perfusion defects on non-invasive testing
- Cerebral–posterior circulation: severe, recurrent, or persistent vertebrobasilar symptoms

Other indications
- Protection of dialysis arteriovenous fistula
- Protection of axillofemoral bypass
- Protection of axillo-axillary bypass
- Protection of LIMA–coronary bypass

Adapted from references 1 and 39.

Table 5.6   Results of Major Percutaneous Treatment Series for SAD

Author Year	No. Patients/ Lesions	Lesion Type	Procedure Success %	Strategy	Stent Type	Mean Follow-up (mos.)	Restenosis %	CVA or TIA %	Limb/LIMA Embolization %	Access-site Complication	Stent Migration %
Becker 1989	418/423	N/A	92	PTA	N/A	N/A	19	1	1%	N/A	N/A
Trinca 1993	30/30	Stenosis	92	PTA	N/A	34	N/A	0	0	7	N/A
Millaire 1993	50/50	Occlusion Stenosis	90	PTA	N/A	41	14	2	0	4	N/A
Mathias 1993	46/46	Occlusion	83	PTA PTA/stent	Wallstent	33	8	0	0	0	0
Kurnar 1995	27/31	Occlusion Stenosis	100	PTA/stent	Palmaz	N/R	N/R	0	0	6	3
Motarjeme 1996	112/93	Occlusion Stenosis	92	PTA/stent	N/R	60	5.3	1	1	0	N/A
Martinez 1997	17/17	Occlusion	94	PTA/stent	Palmaz Wallstent Strecker	19.4	6	0	0	6	6
Sullivan 1998	66/66	Occlusion Stenosis	94	PTA/stent	Palmaz	12.9	5	0	2	7	3
Körner 1999	37/43	Stenosis	84	PTA	N/A	50	17	9	0	7	N/A
Rodriguez-Lopez 1999	69/69	Occlusion Stenosis	96	PTA/stent	Palmaz Wallstent Strecker	13	10	1.4	0	6	1.4
Al-Mubarak 1999	38/38	Occlusion Stenosis	92	PTA/stent	Palmaz Wallstent	20	6	0	0	0	0
Hadjipetrou 1999	18/18	Occlusion Stenosis	100	PTA/stent	Palmaz	20	3	0	0	1	1
Angle 2003	21/21	Occlusion Stenosis	100	PTA PTA/stent	Wallstent	27	26	1	0	2	0
De Vries 2005	110/110		93	PTA PTA/stent	N/A	34	11	4	2	3	0
Henry 2007	237/237	Occlusion Stenosis	94	PTA/stent	Self and balloon expand-able	65	15	0.6	0.6	N/A	N/A
Patel 2007	170/177	Occlusion Stenosis	98	PTA/stent	N/A	35	15	2	1	2	0

N/A, not available; PTA, percutaneous transluminal angioplasty. Adapted from individual references and tables from references 1, 44, 46, and 47.

shift into the vertebral ostium with compromise of antegrade flow. In addition, the dominance of the ipsilateral vertebral artery and the status of the contralateral vertebral artery will influence the neurological sequelae of any compromise in vertebral artery flow.[1] Pseudo-aneurysms have been successfully treated with covered stents.[43]

The major long-term risk of subclavian artery intervention is restenosis. Stenting appears to have significantly reduced the rate of restenosis, from approximately 15%–20% with angioplasty to 0%–10% with stenting. The treatment for restenosis depends on its etiology. Failure to cover the ostium of the vessel will require angioplasty of the area of restenosis and repeat stenting of the ostium. Inadequate stent expansion may be treated with repeat angioplasty and, sometimes, re-stenting.[1]

In the largest stenting series to date, involving 170 patients, procedural success was achieved in 98% of cases (99% for stenoses and 90% for occlusions). Only one stroke occurred and there were no procedure-related deaths. At 30 months of follow-up, the rate of target vessel revascularization was 15%; primary patency was 83%, and secondary patency was 96%.[44]

For total occlusions, rotational atherectomy has been used successfully.[45]

Figures 5.13 and 5.14 show examples of an upper extremity percutaneous intervention.

Surgical treatment of SAD
Surgical options include axillo-axillary bypass (AAB), carotid-to-subclavian bypass (CSB), subclavian-to-subclavian bypass, aortic-to-subclavian bypass, and carotid-subclavian transposition.

Mingoli et al. reported their results of 26 CSB and 17 AAB procedures. Cumulative 5- and 10-year patency rates were 78.3% and 62.9% for the CSB group and 87.9% for the AAB group. In patients with an associated ipsilateral carotid lesion, 5- and 10-year patency rates were 66.0% and 40.8% for the CSB group and 100% for the AAB group.[48]

Reported surgical complications include stroke, TIA, myocardial infarction, hemorrhage, phrenic nerve palsy, Horner's syndrome, delayed wound healing, infection, graft thrombosis, lung atelectasis, pleural effusions, and chylothorax. Intrathoracic surgery is associated with a higher risk of complications.[10]

Gerbitz et al. reported early complications after open revascularization of the subclavian artery (thrombo-endarterectomy, CSB, aortasubclavian bypass, and bypass between the proximal and distal subclavian artery), which included restenosis with embolus or intimal flap in 11% of patients, vocal cord paralysis in 4.2%, phrenic nerve paralysis in 2.8%, one case of Horner's syndrome, and one pneumothorax. Another patient died 10 days postoperatively due to hemorrhage despite three repeat thoracotomies.[49]

In general, perioperative complication rates average 13%, including stroke in about 3% of patients. Surgical perioperative death rates have been reported to be in the 3%–8% range.[2, 50]

Overall symptom recurrence in recent surgical series is 12%.[10]

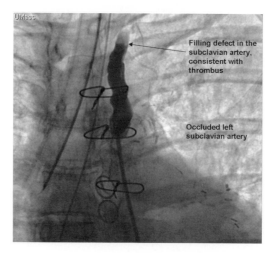

Figure 5.13

Selective angiography showing an occluded left subclavian artery in a patient with prior coronary artery bypass surgery presenting with an ST segment elevation myocardial infarction.

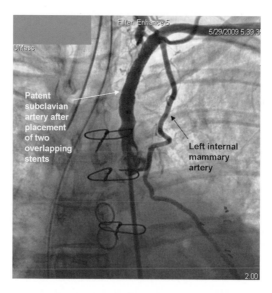

Figure 5.14

Selective angiography reveals a patent left subclavian artery after successful stenting and restored flow in a left internal mammary artery coronary graft.

Other interventional issues

Surgery vs. percutaneous approach Long-term patency appears acceptable after stenting. In a series of 74 patients with subclavian, carotid, or vertebral artery stenosis or occlusion, comparing stenting versus subclavian-to-carotid transposition, 5-year patency rates were similar (95% vs. 100%).[51]

In conclusion, from the available data, surgical revascularization of subclavian stenosis is not a benign procedure, and long-term patency is not significantly better than that of a percutaneous approach. Percutaneous angioplasty and stenting appear to have better outcomes and lower incidence of restenosis when performed for subclavian stenoses than for total chronic occlusions of the subclavian artery, and should be considered as the standard initial approach to subclavian revascularization.

CABG population In patients undergoing CABG, subclavian artery stenting of significant stenoses is an appropriate pre-operative approach and has been performed safely prior to CABG. Similar strategies are used for pre-operative carotid revascularization, with carotid artery stenting prior to CABG (see Chapter VI).[16]

Thoracic outlet syndrome Some authors suggest that asymptomatic patients with cervical or first rib arterial compression should undergo rib resection before the onset of complications from chronic compression.[52]

Treatment for subclavian artery complications of thoracic outlet compression usually involves surgical decompression of the artery (by release of the scalene muscles and removal of any abnormal bony structures) and surgical repair of any structural damage to the artery.[1]

Vasculitis Revascularization in patients with vasculitis is a controversial topic. In the setting of acute vasculitis, medical therapy with immunosuppression is favored, although percutaneous revascularization is indicated if there is impending tissue loss. In the chronic or quiescent phase, revascularization is indicated for symptomatic lesions. Angioplasty or stenting in the setting of vasculitis is thought to be associated with an increased rate of restenosis. Despite the absence of randomized data, the popularity of stent-supported angioplasty in patients with large-vessel vasculitis is increasing.[53, 54]

◇◇◇◇◇◇◇◇◇◇◇

REFERENCES

1. Casserly IP, Kapadia SR. Subclavian artery and upper extremity intervention. In: Bhatt DL, ed. *Guide to Peripheral and Cerebrovascular Intervention.* London: Remedica; 2004.

2. Bonardelli S, Vettoretto N, Tiberio GA, Nodari F, Tardanico R, Giulini SM. Right subclavian artery aneurysms of fibrodysplastic origin: two case reports and review of literature. *J Vasc Surg.* 2001;33:174–177.

3. Ackermann H, Diener HC, Dichgans J. Stenosis and occlusion of the subclavian artery: ultrasonographic and clinical findings. *J Neurol.* 1987;234:396–400.

4. Landry GJ, Liem TK. Endovascular management of Paget-Schroetter syndrome. *Vascular.* 2007;15: 290–296.

5. Brauer RB, Naundorf M, Maurer PC. Surgical and interventional therapeutic possibilities in aneurysms of the subclavian artery. *Zentralbl Chir.* 2000;125:2–6.

6. Phatouros CC, Higashida RT, Malek AM, et al. Endovascular treatment of noncarotid extracranial cerebrovascular disease. *Neurosurg Clin N Am.* 2000;11:331–350.

7. Hashmonai M, Elami A, Kuten A, Lichtig C, Torem S. Subclavian artery occlusion after radiotherapy for carcinoma of the breast. *Cancer.* 1988;61:2015–2018.

8. Gowda AR, Gowda RM, Gowda MR, Khan IA. Takayasu arteritis of subclavian artery in a Caucasian. *Int J Cardiol.* 2004;95:351–354.

9. Das SK, Brow TD, Byrom R. Aortic root anomalies of the neck presenting in adults. Review of the literature with three case reports. *Eur J Vasc Endovasc Surg.* 2005;30:48–51.

10. Hadjipetrou P, Cox S, Piemonte T, Eisenhauer A. Percutaneous revascularization of atherosclerotic obstruction of aortic arch vessels. *J Am Coll Cardiol.* 1999;33:1238–1245.

11. Shadman R, Criqui MH, Bundens WP, et al. Subclavian artery stenosis: Prevalence, risk factors, and association with cardiovascular diseases. *J Am Coll Cardiol.* 2004;44:618–623.

12. Gutierrez GR, Mahrer P, Aharonian V, Mansukhani P, Bruss J. Prevalence of subclavian artery stenosis in patients with peripheral vascular disease. *Angiology.* 2001;52:189–194.

13. Sullivan TM, Gray BH, Bacharach JM, et al. Angioplasty and primary stenting of the subclavian, innominate, and common carotid arteries in 83 patients. *J Vasc Surg.* 1998;28:1059–1065.

14. Al-Mubarak N, Liu MW, Dean LS, et al. Immediate and late outcomes of subclavian artery stenting. *Catheter Cardiovasc Interv.* 1999;46:169–172.

15. Rodriguez-Lopez JA, Werner A, Martinez R, Torruella LJ, Ray LI, Diethrich EB. Stenting for atherosclerotic occlusive disease of the subclavian artery. *Ann Vasc Surg.* 1999;13:254–260.

16. Prasad A, Prasad A, Varghese I, Roesle M, Banerjee S, Brilakis ES. Prevalence and treatment of proximal left subclavian artery stenosis in patients referred for coronary artery bypass surgery. *Int J Cardiol.* 2009;133:109–111.

17. Ringelstein EB, Zeumer H. Delayed reversal of vertebral artery blood flow following percutaneous transluminal angioplasty for subclavian steal syndrome. *Neuroradiology.* 1984;26:189–198.

18. Lobato EB, Kern KB, Bauder-Heit J, Hughes L, Sulek CA. Incidence of coronary-subclavian steal syndrome in patients undergoing noncardiac surgery. *J Cardiothoracic Vasc Anesth.* 2001;15:689–692.

19. Aboyans V, Criqui MH, McDermott MM, et al. The vital prognosis of subclavian stenosis. *J Am Coll Cardiol.* 2007;49:1540–1545.

20. Moran KT, Zide RS, Persson AV, Jewell ER. Natural history of subclavian steal syndrome. *Am Surg.* 1988;54:643–644.

21. Sun Y, Yip PK, Jeng JS, Hwang BS, Lin WH. Ultrasonographic study and long-term follow-up of Takayasu's arteritis. *Stroke.* 1996;27:2178–2182.

22. Subramanyan R, Joy J, Balakrishnan KG. Natural history of aortoarteritis (Takayasu's disease). *Circulation.* 1989;80:429–437.

23. Hirsch AT, Haskal ZJ, Hertzer NR, et al. ACC/AHA 2005 Practice Guidelines for the management of patients with peripheral arterial disease (lower extremity, renal, mesenteric, and abdominal aortic): a collaborative report from the American Association for Vascular Surgery/Society for Vascular Surgery, Society for Cardiovascular Angiography and Interventions, Society for Vascular Medicine and Biology, Society of Interventional Radiology, and the ACC/AHA Task Force on Practice Guidelines (Writing Committee to Develop Guidelines for the Management of Patients with Peripheral Arterial Disease): Endorsed by the American Association of Cardiovascular and Pulmonary Rehabilitation; National Heart, Lung, and Blood Institute; Society for Vascular Nursing; TransAtlantic

Inter-Society Consensus; and Vascular Disease Foundation. *Circulation.* 2006;113:e463–e654.

24. Ackermann H, Diener HC, Seboldt H, Huth C. Ultrasonographic follow-up of subclavian stenosis and occlusion: natural history and surgical treatment. *Stroke.* 1988;19:431–435.

25. Chobanian AV, Bakris GL, Black HR, et al. The seventh report of the Joint National Committee on Prevention, Detection, Evaluation, and Treatment of High Blood Pressure: the JNC 7 report. *JAMA.* 2003;289:2560–2572.

26. English JA, Carell ES, Guidera SA, Tripp HF. Angiographic prevalence and clinical predictors of left subclavian stenosis in patients undergoing diagnostic cardiac catheterization. *Catheter Cardiovasc Interv.* 2001;54:8–11.

27. Osborn LA, Vernon SM, Reynolds B, Timm TC, Allen K. Screening for subclavian artery stenosis in patients who are candidates for coronary bypass surgery. *Catheter Cardiovasc Interv.* 2002;56:162–165.

28. Baxter BT, Blackburn D, Payne K, Pearce WH, Yao JS. Noninvasive evaluation of the upper extremity. *Surg Clin North Am.* 1990;70:87–97.

29. Kalaria VG, Jacob S, Irwin W, Schainfeld RM. Duplex ultrasonography of vertebral and subclavian arteries. *J Am Soc Echocardiogr.* 2005;18:1107–1111.

30. Huang BY, Castillo M. Radiological reasoning: Extracranial causes of unilateral decreased brain perfusion. *AJR Am J Roentgenol.* 2007;189:S49–S54.

31. Hollingworth W, Nathens AB, Kanne JP, et al. The diagnostic accuracy of computed tomography angiography for traumatic or atherosclerotic lesions of the carotid and vertebral arteries: a systematic review. *Eur J Radiol.* 2003;48:88–102.

32. Alegret RE, Blandon RJ, Kirsch J. Poor left internal mammary artery opacification on coronary CT angiography: an indirect sign of subclavian steal. *J Vasc Interv Radiol.* 2008;19:1791–1792.

33. Peloschek P, Sailer J, Loewe C, Schillinger M, Lammer J. The role of multi-slice spiral CT angiography in patient management after endovascular therapy. *Cardiovasc Intervent Radiol.* 2006;29:756–761.

34. Kumar S, Roy S, Radhakrishnan S, Gujral R. Three-dimensional time-of-flight MR angiography of the arch of aorta and its major branches: a comparative study with contrast angiography. *Clin Radiol.* 1996;51:18–21.

35. Okumura A, Araki Y, Nishimura Y, et al. The clinical utility of contrast-enhanced 3D MR angiography for cerebrovascular disease. *Neurol Res.* 2001;23:767–771.

36. Randoux B, Marro B, Koskas F, Chiras J, Dormont D, Marsault C. Proximal great vessels of aortic arch: comparison of three-dimensional gadolinium-enhanced MR angiography and digital subtraction angiography. *Radiology.* 2003;229:697–702.

37. Kumar K, Dorros G, Bates MC, Palmer L, Mathiak L, Dufek C. Primary stent deployment in occlusive subclavian artery disease. *Cathet Cardiovasc Diagn.* 1995;34:281–285.

38. Rogers JH, Calhoun RF, 2nd. Diagnosis and management of subclavian artery stenosis prior to coronary artery bypass grafting in the current era. *J Card Surg.* 2007;22:20–25.

39. Schillinger M, Haumer M, Schillinger S, Mlekusch W, Ahmadi R, Minar E. Outcome of conservative versus interventional treatment of subclavian artery stenosis. *J Endovasc Ther.* 2002;9:139–146.

40. Ferrara F, Meli F, Raimondi F, et al. Subclavian stenosis/occlusion in patients with subclavian steal and previous bypass of internal mammary interventricular anterior artery: medical or surgical treatment? *Ann Vasc Surg.* 2004;18:566–571.

41. Wittwer T, Wahlers T, Dresler C, Haverich A. Carotid-subclavian bypass for subclavian artery revascularization: long-term follow-up and effect of antiplatelet therapy. *Angiology.* 1998;49:279–287.

42. Broadbent LP, Moran CJ, Cross DT, 3rd, Derdeyn CP. Management of ruptures complicating angioplasty and stenting of supraaortic arteries: report of two cases and a review of the literature. *AJNR Am J Neuroradiol.* 2003;24:2057–2061.

43. Schmitter SP, Marx M, Bernstein R, Wack J, Semba CP, Dake MD. Angioplasty-induced subclavian artery dissection in a patient with internal mammary artery graft: treatment with endovascular stent and stent-graft. *AJR Am J Roentgenol.* 1995;165:449–451.

44. Patel SN, White CJ, Collins TJ, et al. Catheter-based treatment of the subclavian and innominate arteries. *Catheter Cardiovasc Interv.* 2008;71:963–968.

45. Martinez R, Rodriguez-Lopez J, Torruella L, Ray L, Lopez-Galarza L, Diethrich EB. Stenting for occlusion of the subclavian arteries. Technical aspects and follow-up results. *Tex Heart Inst J.* 1997;24:23–27.

46. Henry M, Henry I, Polydorou A, Polydorou A, Hugel M. Percutaneous transluminal angioplasty of the subclavian arteries. *Int Angiol.* 2007;26:324–340.

47. Motarjeme A. Percutaneous transluminal angioplasty of supra-aortic vessels. *J Endovasc Surg.* 1996;3:171–181.

48. Mingoli A, Feldhaus RJ, Farina C, Schultz RD, Cavallaro A. Comparative results of carotid-subclavian bypass and axillo-axillary bypass in patients

with symptomatic subclavian disease. *Eur J Vasc Surg.* 1992;6:26–30.

49. Gerbitz J, Braun A, von Segesser LK, Weber E, Turina M. Early results of surgical revascularization of the subclavian artery. *Helv Chir Acta.* 1993;60:171–175.

50. White CJ. Non-surgical treatment of patients with peripheral vascular disease. *Br Med Bull.* 2001;59: 173–192.

51. Linni K, Ugurluoglu A, Mader N, Hitzl W, Magometschnigg H, Holzenbein TJ. Endovascular management versus surgery for proximal subclavian artery lesions. *Ann Vasc Surg.* 2008;22:769–775.

52. Urschel HC, Jr, Razzuk MA. Neurovascular compression in the thoracic outlet: changing management over 50 years. *Ann Surg.* 1998;228:609–617.

53. Sharma BK, Jain S, Bali HK, Jain A, Kumari S. A follow-up study of balloon angioplasty and de-novo stenting in Takayasu arteritis. *Int J Cardiol.* 2000;75(Suppl 1):S147.

54. Bali HK, Jain S, Jain A, Sharma BK. Stent supported angioplasty in Takayasu arteritis. *Int J Cardiol.* 1998;66(Suppl 1):S213.

CHAPTER 6

Carotid Artery Disease

ANATOMY

In normal anatomy, the brachiocephalic, left common carotid, and left subclavian arteries arise from the superior surface of the aortic arch (Figure 6.1).

The aortic arch is classified into three types, based on the relationship of the innominate artery to the aortic arch (Figures 6.2–6.5).[1] The Type I aortic arch is characterized by origin of all 3 great vessels in the same horizontal plane as the outer curvature of the aortic arch. In the Type II aortic arch, the innominate artery originates between the horizontal planes of the outer and inner curvatures of the aortic arch. In the Type III aortic arch, the innominate artery originates below the horizontal plane of the inner curvature of the aortic arch. Type II and III aortic arches are associated with greater technical difficulties with percutaneous interventional procedures of the carotid arteries, due to poor backup support.

The most common anomalies of the great vessels are a common origin of the innominate artery and the left common carotid artery (CCA), and the origin of the left CCA as a separate branch of the innominate artery, also called "bovine configuration" (Figure 6.6 and Table 6.1).

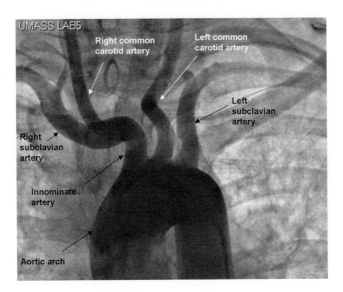

Figure 6.1

Angiography of a normal aortic arch and its major branches.

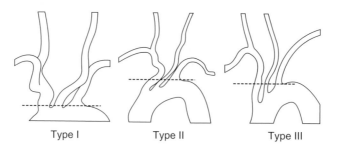

Type I   Type II   Type III

Figure 6.2

Aortic arch types.

Reprinted from: J Am Coll Cardiol, Vol. 49, American College of Cardiology Foundation, American Society of Interventional and Therapeutic Neuroradiology, Society for Cardiovascular Angiography and Interventions, et al. ACCF/SCAI/SVMB/SIR/ASITN 2007 clinical expert consensus document on carotid stenting: a report of the American College of Cardiology Foundation Task Force on Clinical Expert Consensus Documents, Pages 126–70, Copyright, 2007, with permission from Elsevier.

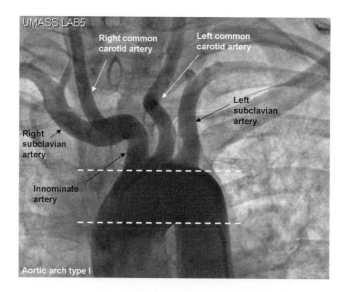

Figure 6.3

Angiogram of a type I aortic arch. The aortic origin of all 3 great vessels is in the same horizontal plane as the outer curvature of the aortic arch (upper dashed line).

The distal CCA usually bifurcates into the internal carotid artery (ICA) and the external carotid artery (ECA) at the level of the thyroid cartilage, but an anomalous bifurcation may occur anywhere within 5 cm above or below this level, and there are many variations in the position of the ICA relative to the ECA.

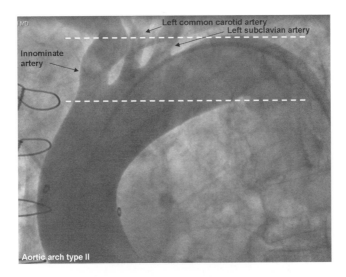

Figure 6.4

Angiography of a type II aortic arch. The innominate artery originates between the horizontal planes of the outer and inner curvatures of the aortic arch (dashed lines).

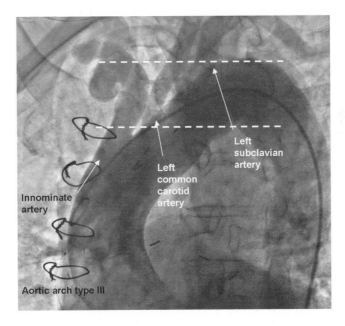

Figure 6.5

Angiogram of a type III aortic arch. The innominate artery originates below the horizontal plane of the inner curvature of the aortic arch (lower dashed line).

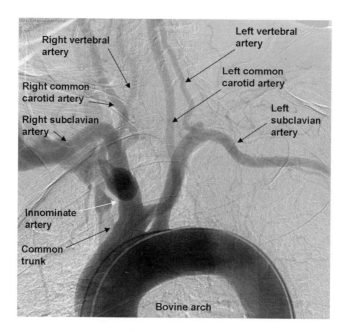

Figure 6.6

Digital substraction angiography of a patient with a bovine arch. The innominate artery and the left common carotid artery share a common trunk.

The dilated origin of the ICA is the carotid bulb, which usually extends 2 cm from the origin, at which point the diameter of the ICA becomes more uniform. There is considerable variation in ICA length and tortuosity, with up to 35% of individuals having some form of undulation, coiling, or kinking of the ICA, particularly the elderly.

The intracranial ICA begins at the skull base where it enters the petrous bone. After passing through the petrous bone in the carotid canal, the ICA transitions into the cavernous segment and eventually enters the subarachnoid space of the brain near the level of the ophthalmic artery. As the ICA turns posteriorly and superiorly, it gives rise to the posterior communicating artery, which communicates with the posterior cerebral artery from the vertebrobasilar circulation. The ICA then bifurcates into the anterior cerebral artery and the middle cerebral artery. The anterior cerebral arteries communicate through the anterior communicating artery. The communicating arteries and their parent segments form the circle of Willis. There are several important cranial collateral pathways, including those from the ECA to the ICA (via the internal maxillary branch of the ECA to the ophthalmic branch of the ICA), ECA to the vertebral artery (via the occipital branch of the ECA), vertebrobasilar system to the ICA (via the posterior communicating artery), and ICA to the ICA (via interhemispheric circulation through the anterior communicating artery). The configuration of the circle of Willis can vary, with a complete circle of Willis being present in fewer than 50% of individuals.

Table 6.1   Anatomical Variants and Anomalies in Cerebral Angiography

Aortic arch

- Innominate and left common carotid artery share common trunk (20%)
- Left common carotid artery originates from innominate artery (bovine arch; 7%)
- Left common carotid artery and left subclavian artery form common trunk (1%)
- Left vertebral artery originates from arch (0.5%; Figure 6.7)
- Aberrant right subclavian artery originates from left side of the arch and passes posterior to esophagus (< 0.5%)

Internal carotid artery

- Location of carotid bifurcation may be T2 to C1
- Absence of internal carotid artery
- Anomalous origin of the internal carotid artery (directly from the arch)
- Hypoplasia of the internal carotid artery
- Duplication of the internal carotid artery
- Anomalous branches of the internal carotid artery (ascending pharyngeal, occipital)
- Aberrant petrous internal carotid artery (course through middle ear)
- Persistent stapedial artery
- Isolated internal carotid artery (fetal origin of the PCA and absent A1 segment)
- Early bifurcation of the middle cerebral artery

Key: PCA, posterior communicating artery. Obtained from reference 1.

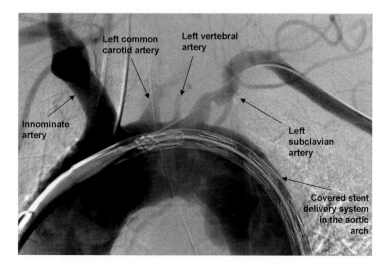

Figure 6.7

Aortic origin of the left vertebral artery.

PHYSIOLOGY AND PATHOPHYSIOLOGY

There are several cardiovascular responses that may occur during carotid manipulation or intervention. Compression or stretching of the carotid sinus can cause a vasovagal (hypotension and bradycardia) or vasodepressor (hypotension without bradycardia) response. These responses are mediated via stimulation of the carotid sinus nerve (a branch of the glossopharyngeal nerve) in the carotid baroreceptor, and vagus nerve activation leading to inhibition of sympathetic tone. The sensitivity of the carotid baroreceptors is variable and may be affected by medications (e.g., vasodilators and beta-blockers may increase sensitivity), the presence of calcified plaque in the carotid bulb (increased sensitivity), or prior carotid endarterectomy (decreased sensitivity).

Although atherosclerosis is the most common disease affecting the carotid circulation (see Chapter 1), other conditions may also be associated with cerebral ischemia and infarction (Table 6.2).

Atherosclerosis in the carotid artery is usually unifocal, with 90% of the lesions located within 2 cm of the ICA origin.

EPIDEMIOLOGY/NATURAL HISTORY

Carotid artery disease is implicated in about a third of all strokes (cerebrovascular accidents [CVAs]). Table 6.3 presents epidemiological points pertaining to stroke, transient ischemic attacks, and carotid artery atherosclerosis.

CLINICAL PRESENTATION

Carotid atherosclerosis can produce retinal and cerebral symptoms by 1 of 2 major mechanisms:

Table 6.2 Causes of Cerebral Ischemia and Infarction

Atherosclerosis
Diseases of the aorta (dissection, aneurysm, aortitis)
Arteritis
Fibromuscular dysplasia
Arterial dissection
Dolichoectasia
Primary vascular tumors
Trauma
Complications of head and neck cancer
Moyamoya's disease

Modified from reference 1.

Table 6.3   Epidemiology of Stroke, TIA, and Carotid Artery Disease

Stroke

- Prevalence
  - Among adults age 20 and older, the prevalence of stroke in 2005 was 6,500,000.

- Incidence
  - Each year about 795,000 people experience a new or recurrent stroke. About 600,000 of these are first attacks, and 185,000 are recurrent attacks.
  - On average, every 40 seconds someone in the United States has a stroke.
  - Men's stroke incidence rates are greater than women's at younger ages but not at older ages. The male/female incidence ratio is 1.25 at ages 55–64, 1.50 for ages 65–74, 1.07 at ages 75–84, and 0.76 at age 85 and older.
  - Blacks have almost twice the risk of first-ever stroke compared with whites.
  - Of all strokes, 87% are ischemic, 10% are intracerebral hemorrhage, and 3% are subarachnoid hemorrhage.

- Mortality
  - Stroke accounted for about 1 of every 17 deaths in the United States in 2005. Stroke mortality for 2005 was 143,579 (56,586 males, 86,993 females).
  - When considered separately from other cardiovascular diseases, stroke ranks No. 3 among all causes of death, behind diseases of the heart and cancer.
  - On average, every 3 to 4 minutes someone dies of a stroke.

- Stroke risk factors
  - The risk of ischemic stroke in smokers is about double that of non-smokers.
  - Atrial fibrillation (AF) is an independent risk factor for stroke, increasing risk about five-fold.
  - High blood pressure is the most important risk factor for stroke. Subjects with blood pressure lower than 120/80 mmHg have about half the lifetime risk of stroke compared to subjects with high blood pressure.
  - A study of over 37,000 women age 45 and older participating in the Women's Health Study suggests that a healthy lifestyle consisting of abstinence from smoking, low body mass index, moderate alcohol consumption, regular exercise, and healthy diet was associated with a significantly reduced risk of total and ischemic stroke but not of hemorrhagic stroke.
  - Among postmenopausal women, the Women's Health Initiative primary prevention clinical trial found that estrogen plus progestin (PremPro) increased ischemic stroke risk by 44%, with no effect on hemorrhagic stroke.

- Physical activity and stroke prevention
  - Physical activity reduces stroke risk. Results from the Physicians' Health Study showed a lower stroke risk associated with vigorous exercise among men (relative risk of total stroke = 0.86 for exercise five times a week or more).

Transient ischemic attacks

- The prevalence of TIA in men is estimated to be 2.7% for ages 65–69 and 3.6% for ages 75–79.
- For women, TIA prevalence is estimated to be 1.6% for ages 65–69 and 4.1% for ages 75–79.
- About 15% of strokes are preceded by a TIA.

Continues

Table 6.3 Epidemiology of Stroke, TIA, and Carotid Artery Disease (Continued)

- About half of patients who experience a TIA fail to report it to their healthcare providers.
- After TIA, the 90-day risk of stroke is 3–17.3%, highest within the first 30 days.
- Within a year of TIA, up to a quarter of patients will die.

Carotid artery disease and stroke

- While extracranial carotid disease is more frequent in Caucasians, intracranial disease is more frequent in African Americans, Hispanics, and Asians.
- Carotid occlusive disease amenable to revascularization accounts for 5% to 12% of new strokes.
- The pattern of progression of carotid stenosis is unpredictable, and disease may progress swiftly or slowly, or remain stable for many years.
- Nearly 80% of strokes due to embolization in the carotid distribution may occur without warning, emphasizing the need for careful patient follow-up.
- The degree of carotid stenosis is associated with stroke risk.

Adapted from references 1 and 2.

- Progressive carotid stenosis leading to in-situ occlusion and hypoperfusion (less common)
- Intracranial arterial occlusion resulting from embolization (more common)

Patients with and without carotid stenosis may develop symptomatic cerebral hypoperfusion from systemic causes. Patients presenting with carotid distribution cerebral ischemia should be thoroughly evaluated for treatable causes, including sources of emboli from the carotid arteries, heart, and aortic arch.

Tables 6.4, 6.5, and 6.6 describe the clinical presentation of some of the most frequent cerebral ischemic syndromes.

Transient ischemic attacks (TIAs) are medical emergencies, characterized by temporary focal retinal and/or hemispheric neurological deficits that resolve within 24 hours. Eleven percent of patients develop a stroke within 90 days after a TIA, one-half occurring within the first 2 days.[4] Patients with both retinal and hemispheric symptoms

Table 6.4 Clinical Syndromes Associated with Extracranial Carotid Occlusive Disease

Retinal syndromes

- TIA
  - Amaurosis fugax or transient monocular blindness
  - Amaurosis fugax variants
- Retinal infarction
  - Central retinal artery occlusion
  - Branch retinal artery occlusion
- Anterior ischemic optic neuropathy

Continues

Table 6.4 Clinical Syndromes Associated with Extracranial Carotid Occlusive Disease (Continued)

Hemispheric syndromes

- TIA
  - Transient hemisphere attack
  - Limb-shaking TIA
- Infarction (stroke)
  - Watershed infarction
  - Thromboembolic stroke

Global cerebral syndromes

- Bilateral or alternating TIAs
- Bilateral simultaneous TIA, suggesting vertebrobasilar insufficiency
- Bilateral cerebral infarction

Key: TIA, transient ischemic attack. Adapted from reference 1.

Table 6.5 Clinical Manifestation Associated with Internal Carotid Artery Branch Occlusion

OCCLUDED ARTERY	CLINICAL MANIFESTATION
Ophthalmic artery	Transient monocular blindness.
Anterior choroidal artery	Contralateral dense hemiparesis: face, arm, leg. Contralateral hemisensory loss (if lateral geniculate is involved, a contralateral hemianopsia).
Recurrent artery of heubner	Mild weakness in the contralateral limb with dysarthria. Abulia with apathy and inertia of movement.
Anterior cerebral artery	Contralateral weakness of the legs and shoulder. Cortical sensory deficit with poor touch localization and extinction with bilateral stimuli (left arm apraxia only).
MCA-M1 segment	Contralateral spastic hemiplegia, visual deficit.
MCA-M2 segment	Hemiparesis affecting the face and arm more than the legs. Visual deficits.
Left hemisphere MCA (superior branch)	Motor aphasia (Broca's aphasia). Also apraxia—both upper extremities. Oral buccal apraxia.
Left hemisphere MCA (inferior branch)	Receptive aphasia (Wernicke's). Non-dominant hemisphere superior MCA Neglect—left side of space. Apraxia in left upper extremity only.
Non-dominant hemisphere inferior MCA	Constructional apraxia and difficulty with shape. Confusion and delirium.

Key: MCA, middle cerebral artery. Adapted from reference 3.

Table 6.6   Clinical Manifestation Associated with Vertebral Artery or Basilar Artery Branch Occlusion

Occluded Artery	Clinical Manifestation
Vertebral artery	
Vertebral or anterior spinal artery	Tongue weakness, weakness of arm and leg, decreased vibration, proprioception, and/or light touch
Vertebral or posterior inferior cerebellar artery	Periorbital and/or facial pain, facial numbness, ataxia of limbs and gait, horizontal nystagmus, tonic gaze deviation, torsional nystagmus, diplopia, vertigo, nausea, vomiting, Horner's syndrome, hoarseness, dysphagia, decreased gag, decreased taste, body numbness, hiccups
Proximal paramedian basilar artery branch	Slow or absent saccades, ataxia of limbs and gait; weakness of abduction; peripheral facial palsy; weakness of arm, leg, and/or face; decreased vibration; proprioception and/or light touch; internuclear ophthalmoplegia
Anterior inferior cerebellar artery	Vertical or horizontal nystagmus, vertigo, nausea, vomiting, sensorineural deafness, tinnitus, slow or absent saccades, ataxia of limbs and gait, peripheral facial palsy, periorbital and/or facial pain, facial numbness, Horner's syndrome, body numbness
Paramedian midbasilar artery	Ataxia of limbs and gait; internuclear ophthalmoplegia; weakness of arm, leg, and/or face; decreased body vibration; proprioception; and/or light touch
Short circumferential midbasilar artery	Ataxia of limbs and gait, decreased facial vibration, proprioception and/or light touch, facial numbness, weak corneal reflex, Horner's syndrome, body numbness, chin deviates to side of lesion with jaw opening
Paramedian distal basilar artery	Ataxia of limbs and gait; internuclear ophthalmoplegia; weakness of arm, leg, and/or face; decreased body vibration; proprioception; and/or light touch
Superior cerebellar artery	Ataxia of limb and gait, horizontal nystagmus, vertigo, nausea, vomiting, Horner's syndrome, body numbness, decreased body vibration, proprioception, and/or light touch
Paramedian terminal basilar artery or proximal posterior cerebral artery	Dilated pupil; ptosis; isotropic and internuclear ophthalmoplegia; weakness of arm, leg, and/or face; hemiataxia and/or hemichorea; tremor; slow or absent saccades; vertical gaze palsy; tonic downgaze; light-near dissociation; skew deviation and corectopia; confusion; disturbance of consciousness
Short circumferential branches of posterior cerebral or posterior communicating artery	Dilated pupil; ptosis; exohypotropia with preserved abduction; intortion; Horner's syndrome; body numbness; hemiataxia; hemichorea; tremor; decreased body vibration;

Continues

Table 6.6   Clinical Manifestation Associated with Vertebral Artery or Basilar Artery Branch Occlusion (Continued)

OCCLUDED ARTERY	CLINICAL MANIFESTATION
	proprioception and/or light touch; weakness of arm, leg, and/or face; skew deviation and corectopia; confusion; disturbance; or consciousness
Posterior cerebral artery	
Ventrolateral artery	Contralateral numbness and tingling, pain, mild contralateral weakness
Posterior communicating artery	Dysphasia in left-sided infarct, hemineglect and impaired visuospatial processing in right sided Infarcts, minor and transient contralateral motor signs
Posterior choroidal artery	Partial hemianopsia
Paramedian artery	Transient loss of consciousness or somnolence, similar to tuberothalamic artery, confusion, amnesia, confabulation if bilateral (thalamic dementia)

Adapted from reference 3.

usually have severe extracranial carotid disease. Rarely, patients with bilateral high-grade ICA stenoses or occlusion may have transient bilateral hemispheric symptoms, which may be mistaken for vertebrobasilar insufficiency.

DIAGNOSTIC EVALUATION

Physical Exam

The physical exam should assess the circulatory system as a whole, with emphasis on the neurovascular system.

A careful history is required to determine whether symptoms are attributable to carotid stenosis. Transient monocular blindness is classically described as a shade coming down over one eye. Hemispheric symptoms include unilateral motor weakness, sensory loss, speech or language disturbances, or visual field disturbances. Vertebrobasilar symptoms include brain stem symptoms (dysarthria, diplopia, dysphagia); cerebellar symptoms (limb or gait ataxia); and simultaneous motor, sensory, and visual loss, which may be unilateral or bilateral. It is important to distinguish between hemispheric and vertebrobasilar symptoms, since patients may have vertebrobasilar insufficiency and asymptomatic carotid stenosis. Accurate localization of symptoms will greatly assist with clinical management and timing of revascularization, if appropriate.

A complete neurological assessment includes the cardiovascular examination (auscultation of the neck for carotid bruits and transmitted murmurs), fundoscopic examination (to detect retinal embolization), and a focused neurologic examination (to correlate neurological symptoms with an ischemic territory). For example, aphasia usually localizes to the left hemisphere, irrespective of the patient's handedness, and hemispatial neglect in the setting of left motor, sensory, or visual signs indicates a right hemisphere lesion.

The sensitivity and specificity of a carotid bruit ranges from 0.29 to 0.75 and 0.61 to 0.88, respectively, to detect carotid stenosis > 50%.[5]

The National Institutes of Health Stroke Scale (NIHSS) is used to quantify the neurological deficit and predict outcome after ischemic stroke (Table 6.7).[6] The NIHSS measures several aspects of brain function including consciousness, vision, sensation, movement, speech, and language. A certain number of points are given for each impairment uncovered during a focused neurological examination. A maximal score of 42 represents the most severe stroke.

The level of stroke severity as measured by the NIH stroke scale scoring system:

0 = no stroke
1–4 = minor stroke
5–15 = moderate stroke
15–20 = moderate/severe stroke
21–42 = severe stroke

Clinical findings must be correlated with brain and vascular imaging to determine whether or not a carotid stenosis is symptomatic.

Imaging is critical to assess the anatomy and structural pathology of the brain (e.g., mass, old or new stroke, hemorrhage, atrophy, or other confounding disease

Table 6.7   National Institutes of Health Stroke Scale

I. a. Level of Consciousness (LOC)	Alert	0
	Drowsy	1
	Stuporous	2
	Coma	3
I. b. LOC Questions	Answers both correctly	0
	Answers one correctly	1
	Incorrect	2
I. c. LOC Commands	Obeys both correctly	0
	Obeys one correctly	1
	Incorrect	2
2. Pupillary Response	Both reactive	0
	One reactive	1
	Neither reactive	2
3. Best Gaze	Normal	0
	Partial gaze palsy	1
	Forced deviation	2

Continues

Table 6.7   National Institutes of Health Stroke Scale (Continued)

4. Best Visual	No visual loss	0
	Partial hemianopia	1
	Complete hemianopia	2
5. Facial Palsy	Normal	0
	Minor	1
	Partial	2
	Complete	3
6. Best Motor Arm	No drift	0
	Drift	1
	Can't resist gravity	2
	No effort against gravity	3
7. Best Motor Leg	No drift	0
	Drift	1
	Can't resist gravity	2
	No effort against gravity	3
8. Plantar Reflex	Normal	0
	Equivocal	1
	Extensor	2
	Bilateral extensor	3
9. Limb Ataxia	Absent	0
	Present in upper or lower	1
	Present in both	2
10. Sensory	Normal	0
	Partial loss	1
	Dense loss	2
11. Neglect	No neglect	0
	Partial neglect	1
	Complete neglect	2
12. Dysarthria	Normal articulation	0
	Mild to moderate dysarthria	1
	Near unintelligible or worse	2
13. Best Language	No aphasia	0
	Mild to moderate aphasia	1
	Severe aphasia	2
	Mute	3
14. Change from Previous Exam	Same	S
	Better	B
	Worse	W
15. Change from Baseline	Same	S
	Better	B
	Worse	W

Adapted from reference 6.

state) and the carotid artery (e.g., anatomic configuration, stenosis, plaque morphology, associated lesions, vasculitis, or dissection), and to guide treatment.

Asymptomatic adults are not recommended to undergo screening for carotid artery stenosis.[7] An exception is a patient scheduled for coronary artery bypass graft surgery (Table 6.8). In patients with asymptomatic carotid bruits, diagnostic tests for carotid disease should only be performed in those patients who are also considered good candidates for carotid revascularization.[1]

Carotid Duplex Ultrasound

Carotid duplex uses spectral Doppler, color flow Doppler, and B-mode ultrasound imaging to evaluate the cervical carotid arteries from their supraclavicular origin to their entrance into the skull base (Figure 6.8).

The mainstay of carotid duplex evaluation is the determination of flow velocity using spectral Doppler analysis. Color-encoded imaging assists in assessment of stenosis severity in individuals with carotid tortuosity, where angle-corrected velocities can be unattainable, and may allow detection of residual flow in patients with subtotal occlusions or vascular calcification.[9, 10]

B-mode imaging is used to identify sites for more focused Doppler evaluation, to directly evaluate cross-sectional narrowing, and to provide information regarding plaque morphology predictive of stroke risk, including surface irregularity, ulceration, and echolucency.[11–13] B-mode may also be useful in measuring intima-media thickness, a marker of systemic atherosclerotic burden and cardiovascular risk used in trials assessing primary risk intervention strategies.[14]

Diagnostic criteria for carotid duplex rely on peak systolic and end-diastolic velocities in the ICA and CCA, spectral patterns, and ICA/CCA velocity ratios. There are numerous diagnostic criteria for grading stenosis severity. A multidisciplinary consensus conference suggests that peak systolic velocity is the single most accurate duplex parameter for determination of stenosis severity.[15]

Compared with angiography, carotid duplex scanning has a sensitivity of 77%–98% and a specificity of 53%–82% to identify or exclude an ICA stenosis greater than or

Table 6.8   Recommended Carotid Stenosis Screening for Patients Undergoing Coronary Artery Bypass Graft Surgery

Age > 65 years
Left main coronary artery disease
Peripheral arterial disease
History of smoking
History of transient ischemic attack
History of stroke
Carotid bruit

Adapted from reference 8.

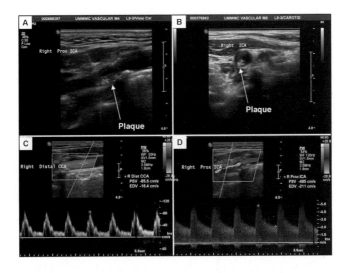

Figure 6.8

Carotid ultrasound in a patient with significant carotid artery stenosis. Panel A: Longitudinal two-dimensional view of the internal carotid artery reveals large heterogeneous plaque burden. Panel B: Transverse two-dimensional view of the same carotid with atherosclerotic plaque. Panel C: Color and spectral Doppler of the distal common carotid artery (proximal to the stenotic segment) reveal laminar blood flow and normal flow velocity. Panel D: Color Doppler of the proximal right internal carotid artery reveals color aliasing suggestive of turbulent flow; spectral Doppler shows an increased velocity of 4.8 meters per second, and a persistent diastolic flow gradient, consistent with severe carotid stenosis. **See Plate 7 for color image.**

Images courtesy of Denise Kush, RDMS, RVT; Vascular Laboratory, UMass Memorial Health Care.

equal to 70%.[16] Women typically have higher flow velocities than men, which may affect decisions about revascularization.[1]

In patients with a severe carotid stenosis or occlusion, compensatory increases in contralateral blood flow may result in high velocities in the contralateral ICA. In this situation, the ICA/CCA velocity ratio (ratio of peak systolic flow velocities in the proximal ICA and the distal CCA) is a better determinant of stenosis severity.[17]

Cardiac arrhythmias, arterial kinking, extensive calcification, high bifurcation, or unusual pathology (e.g., fibromuscular dysplasia or dissection) may impair image interpretation. Lesions in the intracranial ICA and aortic arch cannot be assessed with this technique. When the results of carotid duplex imaging are unclear, diagnostic accuracy may increase to greater than 90% when it is used in conjunction with CTA and/or MRA.[18]

Transcranial Doppler (TCD), with or without color coding, measures intracranial blood-flow patterns and indirectly assesses the effects of stenoses proximal or distal to the assessed sites. It is particularly useful for assessment of intracranial stenoses. Although TCD alone is rarely useful for diagnosis of cervical carotid stenosis, when used as an adjunct to carotid duplex sensitivity, is about 90%. The clinical role for TCD in determining the appropriateness of carotid revascularization remains to be determined.[19]

Magnetic Resonance Angiography

Magnetic resonance angiography (MRA) allows imaging of intrathoracic and intracranial lesions not accessible by carotid duplex. When compared with conventional angiography, first-pass contrast enhanced three-dimensional MRA maximum intensity projections correlate with digital subtraction angiography stenosis in 90% of cases. Interpretability is enhanced by evaluating axial, sagittal, and coronal projections with 3-Tesla magnets (Figure 6.9).[20, 21]

Advantages of MRA include avoidance of nephrotoxic contrast and ionizing radiation. Limitations include the inability to perform MRA due to claustrophobia, pacemakers, implantable defibrillators, and obesity; misdiagnosis of subtotal stenoses as total occlusions; or overestimation of carotid stenoses secondary to movement artifact. These errors may be lessened by using different algorithms or by combining MRA and duplex data. The combination of these two tests provides better concordance with digital subtraction angiography than either test alone (combined 96% sensitivity and 80% specificity) but is not cost effective for routine use.[22]

MRA techniques may allow plaque characterization, including fibrous cap thickness and disruption, and intraplaque lipid content and hemorrhage.[23] MRA does not appear useful for carotid evaluation after stent placement due to artifact.[1]

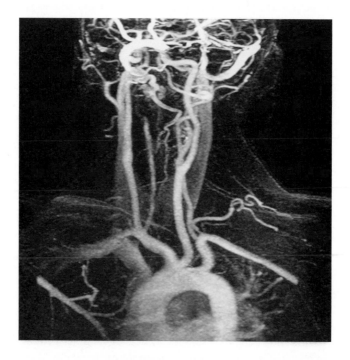

Figure 6.9

Magnetic resonance angiography of the aortic arch, its branches and the carotid circulation.

Figure courtesy of David J. Sheehan, DO; Radiology Department, University of Massachusetts Medical Center and Medical School.

Computed Tomography Angiography

Computed tomography angiography (CTA; Figure 6.10) allows for two-dimensional and three-dimensional reconstructions of the carotid arteries. CTA is useful when carotid duplex is ambiguous, permitting visualization of aortic arch or high bifurcation pathology, reliable differentiation of total and subtotal occlusion, assessment of ostial and tandem stenoses, and evaluation of carotid disease in patients with arrhythmias, valvular heart disease, or cardiomyopathy. Since CTA relies on the recognition of contrast filling of the stenotic vessel lumen, it is less prone to overestimate stenosis severity due to turbulence and arterial tortuosity. CTA has the disadvantage of using nephrotoxic contrast and ionizing radiation.

Although CTA is extremely sensitive to the presence of calcification, it is less reliable than carotid duplex or MRA for assessing plaque vulnerability. When compared with carotid duplex, CTA is more specific for high-grade lesions. When compared with enhanced MRA, one study showed that CTA was less reliable.[24]

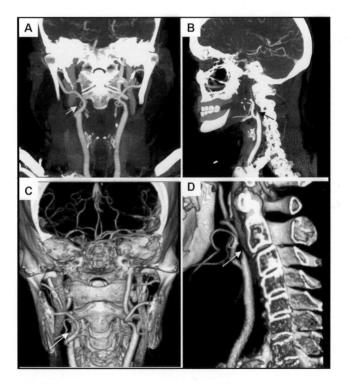

Figure 6.10

Computed tomography angiography in a patient with right internal carotid artery occlusion. Panel A: Coronal two-dimensional maximum intensity projection (MIP) view. Panel B: Sagittal two-dimensional MIP view. Panel C: Coronal three-dimensional reconstruction. Panel D: Sagittal three-dimensional reconstruction. Arrows indicate site of occlusion of the right internal carotid artery. **See Plate 8 for color image**.

Figures courtesy of David J. Sheehan, DO; Radiology Department, University of Massachusetts Medical Center and Medical School.

With CTA, the sensitivity and specificity for detecting carotid stenosis greater than 70% was 85%–95% and 93%–98%, respectively.[25, 26] CTA sensitivity and accuracy can be increased by examining axial source images and volume-rendered projections, and by use of faster high-resolution multislice scanners.[1]

Carotid Angiography

Carotid angiography remains the gold standard for the evaluation of carotid artery disease. As single-plane angiography may underestimate the tortuosity of the vessels, orthogonal, biplane, or rotational angiography is preferred.

The goals of angiography are to define the aortic arch type, configuration of the great vessels, presence of tortuosity and atherosclerotic disease, and other important information (aneurysms, arteriovenous malformations, collateral flow, etc.). This information will influence choice of catheters and interventional strategy (Figure 6.11).

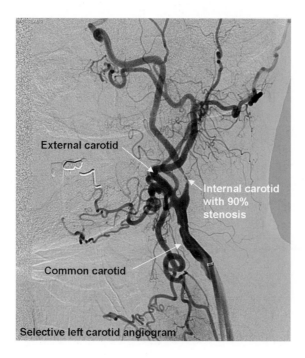

Figure 6.11

Digital substraction selective left carotid angiography in a patient with a 90% internal carotid stenosis.

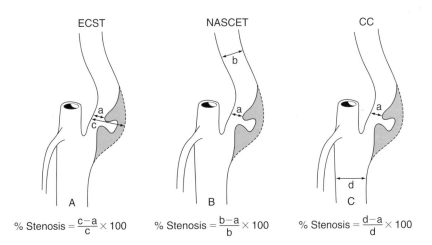

ECST

NASCET

CC

$$\% \text{ Stenosis} = \frac{c-a}{c} \times 100$$

$$\% \text{ Stenosis} = \frac{b-a}{b} \times 100$$

$$\% \text{ Stenosis} = \frac{d-a}{d} \times 100$$

Figure 6.12

Angiographic methods for determining carotid stenosis severity. CC, common carotid; ECST, European Carotid Surgery Trial; NASCET, North American Symptomatic Carotid Endarterectomy Trial.

There are three methods for assessment of carotid stenosis severity, and each relies on different reference segments, resulting in different estimates of stenosis severity (Figure 6.12). By convention, the North American Symptomatic Carotid Endarterectomy Trial (NASCET) method has been adopted, utilizing the diameter of the proximal ICA above the carotid bulb as the reference diameter. Although decisions about the need for carotid endarterectomy (CEA) are often made based on noninvasive imaging, all patients being considered for carotid artery stenting (CAS) must undergo angiography. In these patients, the NASCET definition for stenosis severity should be used, irrespective of estimates of stenosis severity by noninvasive methods.

Carotid angiography shares the same potential complications with other angiographic techniques, including access-site injury, blood transfusion, contrast nephropathy, anaphylactoid reactions, and atheroembolism. In patients with symptomatic cerebral atherosclerosis undergoing diagnostic cerebral angiography, the risk of stroke is 0.5%–5.7%, and the risk of TIA is 0.6%–6.8%.[27] In asymptomatic patients in the ACAS trial, stroke occurred in 1.2% of patients after angiography.[28] More recent studies report neurological complication rates of less than 1%, possibly due to improved technique, catheters, and the use of heparin.[29]

THERAPEUTIC CONSIDERATIONS

Medical Treatment

Risk factor modification

Identification of risk factors for stroke is important for stroke prevention, because modification of many of these risk factors can reduce the risk of stroke. Although not specifically evaluated in patients with severe carotid artery stenosis, cardiovascular risk factor modification and medical therapy are recommended to limit progression of atherosclerosis, irrespective of carotid artery revascularization. Table 6.9 summarizes treatment goals.

- Hypertension. There is a linear relationship between stroke risk and blood pressure. The stroke risk increases three-fold when systolic blood pressure is greater than 160 mmHg. In addition to its detrimental effects on the vasculature, hypertension is also associated with myocardial infarction and atrial fibrillation, both of which

Table 6.9   Summary of Risk Factor Modification Treatment Goals

Risk Factor	Goal	Intervention
Blood pressure	< 140/90 mmHg < 130/80 mmHg with chronic kidney disease or diabetes	Weight control, increased physical activity, alcohol moderation, sodium reduction, medications
Smoking	Smoking cessation Avoid environmental tobacco smoke	Smoking cessation programs, nicotine replacement, bupropion, verenicline
Dyslipidemia	LDL-C < 100 mg/dl (optional goal < 70 mg/dl if high CAD risk) Non-HDL-C < 130 mg/dl	Diet low in saturated fat, weight control, increased physical activity, statins, niacin, fibrates
Diabetes mellitus	HbA1c < 7%	Diet, weight control, oral hypoglycemic agents, insulin
Physical activity	30 minutes, 7 days/week Minimum 5 days/week	Walking, biking, swimming, gardening, household work
Weight management	BMI 18.5–24.9 kg/m^2 Waist circumference: < 40 inches men; < 35 inches women	Physical activity, caloric intake, behavioral programs, rimonabant

Key: BMI, body mass index; CAD, coronary artery disease; HDK-C, high-density lipoprotein cholesterol; LDL-C, low-density lipoprotein cholesterol. Adapted from reference 1.

increase the risk of embolic stroke. Even small reductions in systolic (10 mmHg) and diastolic (3 to 6 mmHg) blood pressure result in a 30%–42% decline in the risk of stroke.[30, 31]

- Smoking Cessation. Cigarette smoking nearly doubles the risk of ischemic and hemorrhagic stroke (particularly subarachnoid hemorrhage), and the risk is directly proportional to the number of cigarettes smoked. The risk is even higher among female smokers who use oral contraceptives. The risk of stroke decreases to that of nonsmokers within 5 years after smoking cessation.[32]
- Dyslipidemia. There is a strong relationship between total dyslipidemia and the extent of extracranial carotid artery atherosclerosis and wall thickness. A meta-analysis of over 70,000 patients at high risk for or with established coronary artery disease showed a 21% relative risk reduction and a 0.9% absolute risk reduction for stroke within 5 years of treatment.[33]
- Diabetes. Diabetics have a two-fold increased risk of stroke when compared with non-diabetics. The combination of diabetes and hypertension increases the risk of stroke six-fold.[1]
- There is an increased risk of stroke in women using oral contraceptives, although most of the risk appears to be concentrated in smokers and women older than 35 years of age.[34]

Pharmacologic therapy
Antiplatelet agents

- All patients with carotid artery disease should be placed on medical therapy, including antiplatelet therapy and other medications, to treat modifiable atherogenic risk factors.
- Asymptomatic patients with one or more risk factors for atherosclerosis should receive antiplatelet therapy for primary prevention of cardiovascular events.
- Symptomatic patients (recent TIA or stroke): The recommendations for antiplatelet therapy are based on large stroke prevention studies that include patients with different stroke etiologies (not only carotid artery disease).[1]
- Aspirin. In primary prevention trials, aspirin decreased the risk of myocardial infarction, but not stroke, in men. In contrast, aspirin appeared to lower the risk of stroke in women.[35]
- Aspirin is the mainstay of secondary prevention in patients with a history of TIA or stroke, with a relative risk reduction of 16% for fatal stroke and 28% reduction in recurrent nonfatal stroke.[36]

- Aspirin is superior to CEA for symptomatic patients with carotid stenosis less than 50% and for asymptomatic patients with carotid stenosis less than 60%.[1]
- There are no data to support the use of aspirin in doses greater than 325 mg daily, even in patients with recurrent TIAs despite low-dose aspirin.
- Dipyridamole is not recommended for primary prevention. Dipyridamole plus aspirin is recommended over aspirin alone for the secondary prevention of stroke.[37]
- Neither ticlopidine nor clopidogrel have been evaluated in primary prevention trials.
- Ticlopidine reduces recurrent stroke by 23% but caused neutropenia in 0.9% of patients in two secondary prevention trials.[38]
- Clopidogrel was similar to aspirin for the secondary prevention of stroke in the CAPRIE trial.[39]
- The combination of aspirin plus clopidogrel was similar in the CHARISMA and the MATCH trials (when compared to aspirin alone in the former and to clopidogrel alone in the latter), but the combination increased the risk of systemic and intracerebral hemorrhage.[40, 41]
- The addition of aspirin to clopidogrel increases the risk of hemorrhage. Combination therapy of aspirin and clopidogrel is not routinely recommended for ischemic stroke or TIA patients unless they have a specific indication for this therapy (i.e., stent or acute coronary syndrome).[37]

Patients who fail antiplatelet therapy

- There are no clinical trials evaluating non-responders who fail antiplatelet therapy.
- Dual antiplatelet therapy is an option in non-responders or those with aspirin or clopidogrel resistance.
- Triple drug therapy with aspirin and clopidogrel plus either aspirin/dipyridamole, cilostazol, or warfarin is an alternative.
- Another option is the addition of warfarin.[1]

Warfarin

- Indicated for both primary and secondary prevention of stroke in patients with atrial fibrillation, to a target International Normalized Ratio (INR) of 2 to 3.
- Warfarin does not appear to be effective in patients with non-cardioembolic stroke: The WARSS and the WASID trials found no difference between warfarin and aspirin in stroke, death, or major bleeding.[42, 43]

Lipid-lowering therapy

- Statins are approved for prevention of stroke in patients with coronary artery disease and may be effective for secondary prevention in patients undergoing CEA.[44]
- In patients without coronary disease, the SPARCL trial studied atorvastatin for the secondary prevention of stroke, with a 16% relative risk reduction.[45]
- The National Cholesterol Education Program guidelines recommend statins in patients with prior TIA or stroke or carotid stenosis greater than 50% stenosis.[46]
- The American Stroke Association also recommends statins for patients with ischemic TIA or stroke.[37]
- Gemfibrozil reduced stroke rates by 24% in the VA-HIT study.[47]
- Niacin reduced stroke by 22% in the Coronary Drug Project.[48]

ACE inhibitors and angiotensin receptor blockers

- In addition to blood pressure reduction, other potential benefits of ACE inhibitors and ARBs include inhibition of angiotensin II–mediated vasoconstriction and vascular smooth cell proliferation, improved endothelial function, and enhanced fibrinolysis.
- The HOPE trial revealed that ramipril 10 mg daily reduced stroke rates by 32% over 5 years, when compared to placebo.[49] The PROGRESS trial showed similar results with perindopril with or without indapamide.[50]
- The LIFE trial evaluated losartan versus atenolol. Although both achieved similar blood pressure reduction, losartan was associated with a 13% reduction in cardiovascular events and a 25% reduction in stroke.[51]

Interventional Treatment

Carotid endarterectomy (CEA)

Indications for and outcomes of CEA have been extensively studied. The support for CEA utilization has been generated from four multicenter, randomized clinical trials comparing surgery versus medical therapy. Table 6.10 summarizes these and other trials.

- The NASCET (North American Symptomatic Carotid Endarterectomy Trial)[52, 53] and ECST (European Carotid Surgery Trial)[54] trials addressed the use of CEA for symptomatic patients with 70%–99% carotid stenosis or selected patients with 50%–69% stenosis.

Table 6.10   Summary of Randomized Trials of CEA Versus Medical Therapy for Carotid Artery Stenosis

TRIAL	N	STENOSIS	FOLLOW-UP (YRS)	END POINT	MEDICAL (%)	CEA (%)	p	RRR (%)	ARR (%)	NNT
Symptomatic										
ECST	3,018	≥ 80%	3	Major stroke or death	26.5	14.9	< 0.001	44	11.6	8.6
NASCET	659	≥ 70%	2	Ipsilateral stroke	26	9	< 0.001	65	17	5.9
VA 309	189	≥ 50%	1	Ipsilateral stroke, TIA, or surgical death	19.4	7.7	0.011	60	11.7	8.5
NASCET	858	50%–69%	5	Ipsilateral stroke	22.2	15.7	0.045	29	6.5	15.4
NASCET	1,368	≤ 50%	5	Ipsilateral stroke	18.7	14.9	0.16	20	3.8	26.3
Asymptomatic										
ACAS	1,662	> 60%	5	Ipsilateral stroke, surgical death	11	5.1	0.004	54	5.9	16.9
ACST	3,120	≥ 60%	5	Any stroke	11.8	6.4	0.0001	46	5.4	18.5
VA	444	≥ 50%	4	Ipsilateral stroke	9.4	4.7	< 0.06	50	4.7	21.3

Key: ACAS, Asymptomatic Carotid Atherosclerotic Study; ACST, Asymptomatic Carotid Surgery Trial; ARR, absolute risk reduction; CEA, carotid endarterectomy; ECST, European Carotid Surgery Trial; NASCET, North American Symptomatic Carotid Endarterectomy Trial; NNT, number needed to treat; RRR, relative risk reduction; TIA, transient ischemic attack; VA, Veterans Affairs. Adapted with information from reference 1.

- The ACAS (Asymptomatic Carotid Atherosclerosis Study)[28] and the ACST (Asymptomatic Carotid Surgery Trial)[55] addressed the use of CEA for asymptomatic patients.
- Limitations of these studies:
  - The general population of patients with carotid stenosis is often different than that of studied patients.
  - NASCET excluded patients older than 80 years of age and high-risk patients with liver, kidney cardiac valvular or rhythm disorders, recent myocardial infarction, uncontrolled hypertension, or diabetes.
  - In asymptomatic patients, the ACAS and ACST had only a 5.4%–5.9% absolute risk reduction of stroke over 5 years. Therefore, if the surgical risk exceeds 3%, no overall benefit may exist. The low complication rates in these highly selected trial populations and high-volume medical centers are not the same as in the general population, with a potential offset of the benefit. Furthermore, a study of Medicare mortality data from hospitals participating in NASCET and ACAS demonstrated a 1.4% perioperative mortality compared with 0.6% reported in NASCET and 0.1% reported in ACAS. Low-volume hospitals can have CEA-related mortality rates of about 2.5%.[56]
  - Medical therapy has improved since these trials. In NASCET, for example, medical therapy was limited to 1300 mg of aspirin daily, a dose that is no longer used. ACE inhibitors, ARBs, and statins are now available.

- Guidelines of the American Heart Association establish an upper limit of 6% for perioperative risk in symptomatic patients and a 3% upper limit in asymptomatic patients, assuming a life expectancy of > 5 years.[57]
- Perioperative stroke and death rates with different comorbidities are:
  - 8.6% for patients with congestive heart failure
  - 7.5% for patients older than 75 years
  - 7.5% for postendarterectomy restenosis
  - 13.9% for ipsilateral carotid siphon stenosis
  - 10%–18% for the presence of intraluminal thrombus
  - 14.3% for contralateral carotid occlusion
  - 16%–26% for CEA combined with coronary artery bypass grafting

Carotid stenting

Multiple trials evaluating carotid stenting are now available. Key characteristics of these trials are described in Table 6.11.

The use of embolic protection devices has been further supported by numerous radiologic studies examining the frequency of ischemic diffusion-weighted magnetic

Table 6.11 Landmark Trials of Endovascular versus Surgical Treatment for Carotid Stenosis

TRIAL	DESIGN	EVALUATION	N	DISTAL PROTECTION	COMMENTS	OUTCOMES
CAVATAS (Carotid and Vertebral Artery Transluminal Angioplasty Study)[57]	Multicenter international RCT	Angioplasty vs. CEA	504	No	Only 26% of patients were stented. High-risk surgical pts. excluded (diabetics, recent MI, poorly controlled HTN, kidney disease, etc.).	No statistical difference in the rate of disabling stroke or death within 30 days (6.4% CAS vs. 5.9% CEA). No significant difference in the 3-year ipsilateral stroke rate.
Wallstent[58, 59]	Multicenter randomized trial	To evaluate CEA and CAS equivalence	219	No	Symptomatic patients with 60% to 99% stenosis. No distal protection devices.	30-day stroke or death rates were 12.1% with CAS and 4.5% with CEA (p = 0.049). Additionally, 12.1% of CAS patients suffered ipsilateral stroke, procedure-related death, or vascular death at 1 year, versus 3.6% of CEA patients (p = 0.022).
CaRESS (Carotid Revascularization Using Endarterectomy or Stenting Systems)[60, 61]	Multicenter, nonrandomized	CAS with embolic protection (N = 143) vs. CEA (N = 254)	397	Yes	Symptomatic (32%) and asymptomatic (68%) patients with low and high surgical risk	No statistically significant difference between 30-day and 1-year death or stroke rates existed between CAS and CEA (2.1% vs. 3.6%, and 10.0% vs. 13.6%, respectively). No significant differences for restenosis, residual stenosis, repeat angiography, and need for repeat carotid revascularization.

Continues

Table 6.11   Landmark Trials of Endovascular versus Surgical Treatment for Carotid Stenosis (Continued)

Trial	Design	Evaluation	N	Distal Protection	Comments	Outcomes
SAPPHIRE (Stenting and Angioplasty with Protection in Patients at High Risk for Endarterectomy)[62]	Randomized, multicenter trial	To determine CAS noninferiority to CEA in high-risk patients	344	Yes	Symptomatic stenosis of at least 50% or asymptomatic stenosis of at least 80%.	The 30-day MI, stroke, or death rate was 4.8% for CAS and 9.8% for CEA (p = 0.09). Much of this difference was secondary to MIs in the CEA group. 30-day rate of stroke and death was 4.8% for CAS patients and 5.6% for CEA patients. At 1 year, 12.2% of CAS patients had suffered stroke, MI, or death versus 20.1% of CEA patients (noninferiority analysis: p = 0.004; superiority analysis: intention-to-treat p = 0.053, as-treated p = 0.048). Myocardial infarction and major ipsilateral stroke rates were significantly better after CAS versus CEA (2.5% vs. 8.1%, p = 0.03; 0% vs. 3.5%, p = 0.02; respectively).
SPACE (Stent-supported Percutaneous Angioplasty of the Carotid artery versus Endarterectomy) trial[63]	Randomized, multicenter	Noninferiority for CAS compared with CEA in patients with low risk	1,183	Not required and was only used in 27% of cases	Symptomatic carotid artery stenosis (70% by duplex ultrasonography, 50% by NASCET criteria, or 70% by ECST criteria)	The 30-day rates of ipsilateral stroke or death were 6.84% for CAS and 6.34% for CEA (p value not significant). Did not prove noninferiority of CAS statistically, because it was underpowered.
EVA-3S (Endarterectomy Versus Angioplasty in Patients with Symptomatic Severe Carotid Stenosis)[64]	Multicenter, randomized trial	Noninferiority of CAS versus CEA in patients with > 60% stenosis	527	Early in the trial, the use of embolic protection was not required. Patients treated without embolic protection experienced a 25% 30-day rate of stroke or death (5 of 20 patients), prompting protocol changes by the EVA-3S safety committee.	Compared groups of physicians with unequal experience. Surgeons performing CEA had performed at least 25 endarterectomies in the year before trial entry, yet endovascular physicians were certified after completing as few as 5 to 12 CAS procedures. Endovascular physicians were also allowed to enroll study patients while simultaneously undergoing training and certification.	Prematurely stopped after rate of any stroke or death was significantly higher in the CAS group (9.6%) than the CEA group (3.9%) (p = 0.01).

resonance imaging lesions in the postoperative period. These studies have demonstrated the following:

- A reduction in the frequency of ischemic lesions with distal embolic protection (49% vs. 67%).[65]
- Fewer ischemic lesions after CEA than with CAS (11.6% vs. 42.6%) with current embolic protection devices.[66]

Table 6.12 compares different types of protection devices.

Carotid artery stent registries help establish the "real world" adverse event rates in high-risk CAS patients. Results of some of these registries are summarized in Table 6.13.

Table 6.12 Comparison of Proximal and Distal Embolic Protection

ADVANTAGES	DISADVANTAGES
Proximal embolic protection with balloon occlusion	
• Transient reversal of flow in distal ICA • Operator can select a guidewire of choice; avoids embolization during initial passage of guidewire and throughout procedure	• More cumbersome to use than other devices; large profile, large sheath size • Imaging during device advancement via stagnant contrast • Arterial occlusion may be poorly tolerated
Distal embolic protection with balloon occlusion	
• Easy to use • Compatible with all stents • Aspirate large and small particles • Reliably trap debris	• No antegrade flow • 2%–5% are intolerant • Balloon-induced injury • Not as steerable as PTCA guidewires • Difficult to image during the procedure • Loss of apposition during procedure
Distal embolic protection with filter devices	
• Preserve antegrade flow • Contrast imaging is possible throughout the procedure • Some devices allow operator to select an independent guidewire to cross target • lesion	• May not capture all debris • Difficult to evaluate retrieval of debris during the procedure • Filters may clog • Delivery/retrieval catheters may cause embolization • Filter entrapment in the stent • Some EPDs are not as steerable as PTCA guidewires

EPD, embolic protection device; ICA, internal carotid artery; PTCA, percutaneous transluminal coronary angioplasty.
Adapted from reference 1.

Table 6.13   Carotid Artery Stent Registries

REGISTRY	N	STENT	EMBOLIC PROTECTION DEVICE	COMMENTS
ARCHeR	581	Acculink	Accunet	30 day MI/stroke/death 8.3% 1 yr stroke/death 9.6%
BEACH	480	Wallstent	FilterWire	30 day MI/stroke/death 5.8% 1 yr MI/stroke/death 9.1%
CABERNET	454	NexStent	FilterWire	30 day MI/stroke/death 3.8% 1 yr MI/stroke/death 4.5%
CAPTURE	2,500	RX Acculink	Accunet	30 day MI/stroke/death 5.7%
CaRESS	143	Wallstent	Guardwire Plus	30 day stroke/death 2.1%
CREATE Pivotal	419	Protege	SPIDER OTW	30 day MI/stroke/death 6.2%
CREATE SpideRx	125	Acculink	SpideRx	30 day MI/stroke/death 5.6%
CREST	749	RX Acculink	RX Accunet	30 day stroke/death 4.4%
MAVErIC I	99	Exponent	GuardWire	30 day MI/stroke/death 5.1%
MAVErIC II	399	Exponent	GuardWire	30 day MI/stroke/death 5.3%
MO.MA	157	Any	MO.MA	30 day stroke/death 5.7%
PRIAMUS	416	Any	MO.MA	30 day stroke/death 4.6%
SECuRITY	398	Xact Carotid Stent	Emboshield	30 day MI/stroke/death 8.5%

ARCHeR, Acculink for Revascularization of Carotids in High-Risk Patients; BEACH, Boston Scientific EPI: A Carotid Stenting Trial for High Risk Surgical Patients; CABERNET, Carotid Artery Revascularization Using Boston Scientific EPI Filterwire EX/EZ and the EndoTex NexStent; CAPTURE, Carotid Acculink/Accunet Post Approval Trial to Uncover Rare Events; CaRESS, Carotid Revascularization using Endarterectomy or Stenting Systems; CREATE, Carotid Revascularization with ev3 Arterial Technology Evaluation; CREST, Carotid Revascularization Endarterectomy versus Stent Trial; MAVErIC, Endarterectomy versus Angioplasty in Patients with Severe Symptomatic Carotid Stenosis; MI, myocardial infarction; MO.MA, Multicenter Registry to Assess the Safety and Efficacy of the MO.MA Cerebral Protection Device During Carotid Stenting; SECuRITY, Registry Study to Evaluate the NeuroShield Bare Wire Cerebral Protection System and X-Act Stent in Patients at High Risk for Carotid Endarterectomy. Table adapted from reference 1.

Figures 6.13 and 6.14 are representative of a typical CAS case.

There are two major ongoing, randomized trials of CAS versus CEA: CREST (Carotid Revascularization Endarterectomy versus Stent Trial) and ICSS (International Carotid Stenting Study).

Optimal treatment selection

Asymptomatic patients   There are multiple controversies regarding the management of asymptomatic patients with carotid artery disease. This is of paramount importance, because asymptomatic patients with carotid stenosis comprise 80%–90% of the population undergoing revascularization.[1]

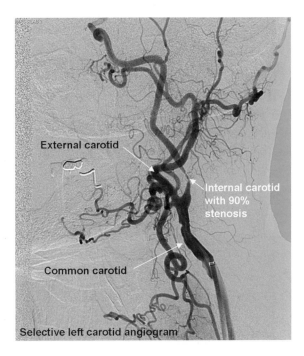

External carotid

Internal carotid with 90% stenosis

Common carotid

Selective left carotid angiogram

Figure 6.13

Digital substraction selective left carotid angiography reveals a 90% internal carotid stenosis prior to intervention.

- Is revascularization an adequate treatment?
  - Favoring revascularization. The ACAS and ACST trials demonstrated superiority of CEA and ASA compared with aspirin alone in patients at low surgical risk.[28, 55]
  - Arguments against revascularization. Aggressive medical therapy has evolved dramatically since these trials were performed, and data from these trials may be outdated.
- What threshold should be used for revascularization?
  - ACAS and ACST concluded that CEA was superior to aspirin in patients with asymptomatic stenosis greater than 60%, but the ACST did not demonstrate difference in the risk of stroke for increasing stenosis severity between 60% and 99% (an issue not evaluated by the ACAS trial). Since the absolute risk reduction of stroke is about 1% per year for CEA compared with aspirin, it is reasonable to wonder whether the threshold for carotid revascularization

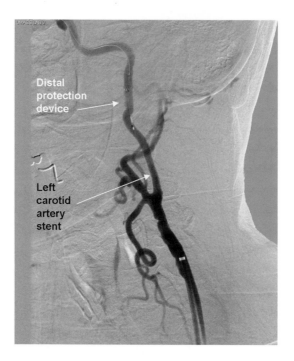

Figure 6.14

Digital substraction selective left carotid angiography after successful stenting. A distal protection device is visualized.

in asymptomatic patients should be increased to 80%. The AHA guidelines address this issue by recommending revascularization in asymptomatic patients with stenosis > 60% and < 75% if the surgical risk is < 3%; asymptomatic patients with stenoses > 75% could be revascularized if the surgical risk is 3%–5%.[68] These same recommendations are provided by the American College of Cardiology Consensus on Carotid Stenting and the Society for Vascular Surgery Guidelines.[1, 69]

- Should carotid duplex imaging results guide the decision to revascularize an asymptomatic patient?
  - This has not been addressed; these trials relied on angiographic assessment.
- Should an asymptomatic low-risk patient be revascularized by CAS or CEA?
  - Randomized clinical trial data supporting low-risk revascularization only exist for CEA. If current trials of CEA versus CAS show equivalence or superiority of CAS, then CAS may become the technique of choice for asymptomatic patients at low risk for CEA.

- Should asymptomatic patients at high risk for CEA be revascularized?
  - ○ These patients were excluded from trials of CEA and medical therapy.
  - ○ There are insufficient data in these high-risk asymptomatic patients to define the natural history with respect to 5-year stroke-free survival.
  - ○ The fact that the benefits of revascularization are negated by the high risk does not mandate that these patients undergo CAS.

Symptomatic patients Recent guidelines for the interventional management of atherosclerotic carotid artery disease by the Society for Vascular Surgery and American Heart Association (Table 6.14) can be summarized as follows:[70]

- Aggressive medical therapy without revascularization is recommended in symptomatic patients with < 50% stenosis.
- Carotid endarterectomy plus medical therapy is recommended in symptomatic patients with > 50% stenosis.
- Carotid stenting is an alternative for patients with severe carotid stenosis and high-risk clinical or anatomic characteristics (Table 6.15).[69]

Therefore, it is reasonable to offer CAS over CEA to patients meeting high-risk criteria (Table 6.15), whether symptomatic or asymptomatic. However, additional characteristics need to be taken into account, as they may predict poor likelihood of stenting success. These factors include the degree of plaque calcification, the complexity of the aortic arch, the tortuosity of the vessels, and the luminal diameter.

Table 6.14 American Heart Association and American Stroke Association Recommendations for Revascularization in Symptomatic Patients with Carotid Artery Stenosis

- For patients with recent TIA or ischemic stroke within the last 6 months and ipsilateral severe (70%–99%) carotid artery stenosis, CEA is recommended by a surgeon with a perioperative morbidity and mortality rate of < 6%.
- For patients with recent TIA or ischemic stroke and ipsilateral moderate (50%–69%) carotid stenosis, CEA is recommended, depending on patient-specific factors such as age, gender, comorbidities, and severity of initial symptoms.
- When degree of stenosis is < 50%, there is no indication for CEA.
- When CEA is indicated, surgery within 2 weeks rather than delayed surgery is suggested.
- Among patients with symptomatic severe stenosis (> 70%) in whom the stenosis is difficult to access surgically, medical conditions are present that greatly increase the risk for surgery, or when other specific circumstances exist such as radiation-induced stenosis or restenosis after CEA, CAS is not inferior to CEA and may be considered.
- CAS is reasonable when performed by operators with established periprocedural morbidity and mortality rates of 4%–6%, similar to that observed in trials of CEA and CAS.

Key: CAS, carotid artery stenting; CEA, carotid endarterectomy; TIA, transient ischemic attack. Table adapted from reference 1.

Table 6.15   High-Risk Criteria—Probably Better Served by Stenting

Anatomical

- Restenosis after CEA
- Contralateral occlusion
- Previous neck radiation or surgery
- Surgically inaccessible lesions (e.g., located above the C-2 level, below the clavicle)
- Neck immobility
- Tracheostomy
- Contralateral laryngeal palsy
- Bilateral severe stenotic lesions requiring treatment
- Severe intracranial stenosis

Medical comorbidities

- Unstable angina
- Poor cardiac ejection fraction
- Congestive heart failure
- Planned coronary artery bypass operation
- Obstructive pulmonary disease
- Advanced age (>75 or 80 years)

Table adapted from reference 69.

◇◇◇◇◇◇◇◇◇◇◇◇◇

REFERENCES

1. American College of Cardiology Foundation, American Society of Interventional and Therapeutic Neuroradiology, Society for Cardiovascular Angiography and Interventions, et al. ACCF/SCAI/SVMB/SIR/ASITN 2007 clinical expert consensus document on carotid stenting: a report of the American College of Cardiology Foundation Task Force on Clinical Expert Consensus Documents (ACCF/SCAI/SVMB/SIR/ASITN Clinical Expert Consensus Document Committee on Carotid Stenting). *J Am Coll Cardiol.* 2007;49:126–170.

2. Writing Group Members, Lloyd-Jones D, Adams R, et al. Heart disease and stroke statistics—2009 update: a report from the American Heart Association Statistics Committee and Stroke Statistics Subcommittee. *Circulation.* 2009;119:e21–e181.

3. Cho L, Mukherjee D. Basic cerebral anatomy for the carotid interventionalist: the intracranial and extracranial vessels. *Catheter Cardiovasc Interv.* 2006;68:104–111.

4. Albers GW, Caplan LR, Easton JD, et al. Transient ischemic attack—proposal for a new definition. *N Engl J Med.* 2002;347:1713–1716.

5. Rea T. The role of carotid bruit in screening for carotid stenosis. *Ann Intern Med.* 1997;127:657–658.

6. Brott T, Adams HP, Jr, Olinger CP, et al. Measurements of acute cerebral infarction: a clinical examination scale. *Stroke.* 1989;20:864–870.

7. U.S. Preventive Services Task Force. Screening for carotid artery stenosis: U.S. Preventive Services Task Force recommendation statement. *Ann Intern Med.* 2007;147:854–859.

8. Eagle KA, Guyton RA, Davidoff R, et al. ACC/AHA 2004 guideline update for coronary artery bypass graft surgery: summary article. A report of the American College of Cardiology/American Heart Association Task Force on Practice Guidelines (Committee to Update the 1999 Guidelines for Coronary Artery Bypass Graft Surgery). *J Am Coll Cardiol.* 2004;44:e213–e310.

9. Bray JM, Galland F, Lhoste P, et al. Colour Doppler and duplex sonography and angiography of the carotid artery bifurcations. Prospective, double-blind study. *Neuroradiology*. 1995;37:219–224.

10. Bluth EI, Sunshine JH, Lyons JB, et al. Power Doppler imaging: initial evaluation as a screening examination for carotid artery stenosis. *Radiology*. 2000;215:791–800.

11. Streifler JY, Eliasziw M, Fox AJ, et al. Angiographic detection of carotid plaque ulceration. Comparison with surgical observations in a multicenter study. North American Symptomatic Carotid Endarterectomy Trial. *Stroke*. 1994;25:1130–1132.

12. Lovett JK, Redgrave JN, Rothwell PM. A critical appraisal of the performance, reporting, and interpretation of studies comparing carotid plaque imaging with histology. *Stroke*. 2005;36:1091–1097.

13. Biasi GM, Froio A, Diethrich EB, et al. Carotid plaque echolucency increases the risk of stroke in carotid stenting: the Imaging in Carotid Angioplasty and Risk of Stroke (ICAROS) study. *Circulation*. 2004;110:756–762.

14. Hodis HN, Mack WJ, LaBree L, et al. The role of carotid arterial intima-media thickness in predicting clinical coronary events. *Ann Intern Med*. 1998;128:262–269.

15. Grant EG, Benson CB, Moneta GL, et al. Carotid artery stenosis: Gray-scale and Doppler US diagnosis—Society of Radiologists in Ultrasound Consensus Conference. *Radiology*. 2003;229:340–346.

16. Sabeti S, Schillinger M, Mlekusch W, et al. Quantification of internal carotid artery stenosis with duplex US: comparative analysis of different flow velocity criteria. *Radiology*. 2004;232:431–439.

17. Busuttil SJ, Franklin DP, Youkey JR, Elmore JR. Carotid duplex overestimation of stenosis due to severe contralateral disease. *Am J Surg*. 1996;172:144–147.

18. Patel MR, Kuntz KM, Klufas RA, et al. Preoperative assessment of the carotid bifurcation. Can magnetic resonance angiography and duplex ultrasonography replace contrast arteriography? *Stroke*. 1995;26:1753–1758.

19. Sloan MA, Alexandrov AV, Tegeler CH, et al. Assessment: transcranial Doppler ultrasonography: Report of the Therapeutics and Technology Assessment Subcommittee of the American Academy of Neurology. *Neurology*. 2004;62:1468–1481.

20. Remonda L, Senn P, Barth A, Arnold M, Lovblad KO, Schroth G. Contrast-enhanced 3D MR angiography of the carotid artery: comparison with conventional digital subtraction angiography. *AJNR Am J Neuroradiol*. 2002;23:213–219.

21. Cosottini M, Pingitore A, Puglioli M, et al. Contrast-enhanced three-dimensional magnetic resonance angiography of atherosclerotic internal carotid stenosis as the noninvasive imaging modality in revascularization decision making. *Stroke*. 2003;34:660–664.

22. Buskens E, Nederkoorn PJ, Buijs-Van Der Woude T, et al. Imaging of carotid arteries in symptomatic patients: cost-effectiveness of diagnostic strategies. *Radiology*. 2004;233:101–112.

23. Yuan C, Mitsumori LM, Ferguson MS, et al. In vivo accuracy of multispectral magnetic resonance imaging for identifying lipid-rich necrotic cores and intraplaque hemorrhage in advanced human carotid plaques. *Circulation*. 2001;104:2051–2056.

24. Wutke R, Lang W, Fellner C, et al. High-resolution, contrast-enhanced magnetic resonance angiography with elliptical centric k-space ordering of supra-aortic arteries compared with selective X-ray angiography. *Stroke*. 2002;33:1522–1529.

25. Hollingworth W, Nathens AB, Kanne JP, et al. The diagnostic accuracy of computed tomography angiography for traumatic or atherosclerotic lesions of the carotid and vertebral arteries: A systematic review. *Eur J Radiol*. 2003;48:88–102.

26. Koelemay MJ, Nederkoorn PJ, Reitsma JB, Majoie CB. Systematic review of computed tomographic angiography for assessment of carotid artery disease. *Stroke*. 2004;35:2306–2312.

27. Connors JJ, 3rd, Sacks D, Furlan AJ, et al. Training, competency, and credentialing standards for diagnostic cervicocerebral angiography, carotid stenting, and cerebrovascular intervention: a joint statement from the American Academy of Neurology, American Association of Neurological Surgeons, American Society of Interventional and Therapeutic Radiology, American Society of Neuroradiology, Congress of Neurological Surgeons, AANS/CNS Cerebrovascular Section, and Society of Interventional Radiology. *Radiology*. 2005;234:26–34.

28. Executive Committee for the Asymptomatic Carotid Atherosclerosis Study. Endarterectomy for asymptomatic carotid artery stenosis. *JAMA*. 1995;273:1421–1428.

29. Fayed AM, White CJ, Ramee SR, Jenkins JS, Collins TJ. Carotid and cerebral angiography performed by cardiologists: cerebrovascular complications. *Catheter Cardiovasc Interv*. 2002;55:277–280.

30. Collins R, Peto R, MacMahon S, et al. Blood pressure, stroke, and coronary heart disease. Part 2, Short-term reductions in blood pressure: overview of randomised drug trials in their epidemiological context. *Lancet*. 1990;335:827–838.

31. Staessen JA, Gasowski J, Wang JG, et al. Risks of untreated and treated isolated systolic hypertension in the elderly: meta-analysis of outcome trials. *Lancet.* 2000;355:865–872.

32. Kawachi I, Colditz GA, Stampfer MJ, et al. Smoking cessation and decreased risk of stroke in women. *JAMA.* 1993;269:232–236.

33. Amarenco P, Lavallee P, Touboul PJ. Stroke prevention, blood cholesterol, and statins. *Lancet Neurol.* 2004;3:271–278.

34. Royal College of General Practitioners' Oral Contraception Study. Further analyses of mortality in oral contraceptive users. *Lancet.* 1981;1:541–546.

35. Ridker PM, Cook NR, Lee IM, et al. A randomized trial of low-dose aspirin in the primary prevention of cardiovascular disease in women. *N Engl J Med.* 2005;352:1293–1304.

36. Antithrombotic Trialists' Collaboration. Collaborative meta-analysis of randomised trials of antiplatelet therapy for prevention of death, myocardial infarction, and stroke in high risk patients. *BMJ.* 2002;324:71–86.

37. Adams RJ, Albers G, Alberts MJ, et al. Update to the AHA/ASA recommendations for the prevention of stroke in patients with stroke and transient ischemic attack. *Stroke.* 2008;39:1647–1652.

38. Hass WK, Easton JD, Adams HP, Jr, et al. A randomized trial comparing ticlopidine hydrochloride with aspirin for the prevention of stroke in high-risk patients. Ticlopidine Aspirin Stroke Study Group. *N Engl J Med.* 1989;321:501–507.

39. CAPRIE Steering Committee. A randomised, blinded, trial of clopidogrel versus aspirin in patients at risk of ischaemic events (CAPRIE). *Lancet.* 1996;348: 1329–1339.

40. Diener HC, Bogousslavsky J, Brass LM, et al. Management of atherothrombosis with clopidogrel in high-risk patients with recent transient ischaemic attack or ischaemic stroke (MATCH): study design and baseline data. *Cerebrovasc Dis.* 2004;17:253–261.

41. Bhatt DL, Fox KA, Hacke W, et al. Clopidogrel and aspirin versus aspirin alone for the prevention of atherothrombotic events. *N Engl J Med.* 2006;354:1706–1717.

42. Mohr JP, Thompson JL, Lazar RM, et al. A comparison of warfarin and aspirin for the prevention of recurrent ischemic stroke. *N Engl J Med.* 2001;345: 1444–1451.

43. Chimowitz MI, Kokkinos J, Strong J, et al. The Warfarin-Aspirin Symptomatic Intracranial Disease Study. *Neurology.* 1995;45:1488–1493.

44. McGirt MJ, Perler BA, Brooke BS, et al. 3-hydroxy-3-methylglutaryl coenzyme A reductase inhibitors reduce the risk of perioperative stroke and mortality after carotid endarterectomy. *J Vasc Surg.* 2005;42: 829–836.

45. Amarenco P, Bogousslavsky J, Callahan A, 3rd, et al. High-dose atorvastatin after stroke or transient ischemic attack. *N Engl J Med.* 2006;355:549–559.

46. Grundy SM, Cleeman JI, Merz CN, et al. Implications of recent clinical trials for the National Cholesterol Education Program Adult Treatment Panel III Guidelines. *J Am Coll Cardiol.* 2004;44:720–732.

47. Rubins HB, Robins SJ, Collins D, et al. Gemfibrozil for the secondary prevention of coronary heart disease in men with low levels of high-density lipoprotein cholesterol. Veterans Affairs High-Density Lipoprotein Cholesterol Intervention Trial Study Group. *N Engl J Med.* 1999;341:410–418.

48. Canner PL, Berge KG, Wenger NK, et al. Fifteen year mortality in Coronary Drug Project patients: long-term benefit with niacin. *J Am Coll Cardiol.* 1986;8:1245–1255.

49. Yusuf S, Sleight P, Pogue J, Bosch J, Davies R, Dagenais G. Effects of an angiotensin-converting-enzyme inhibitor, ramipril, on cardiovascular events in high-risk patients. The Heart Outcomes Prevention Evaluation Study Investigators. *N Engl J Med.* 2000;342:145–153.

50. PROGRESS Collaborative Group. Randomised trial of a perindopril-based blood-pressure-lowering regimen among 6,105 individuals with previous stroke or transient ischaemic attack. *Lancet.* 2001;358: 1033–1041.

51. Dahlof B, Devereux RB, Kjeldsen SE, et al. Cardiovascular morbidity and mortality in the Losartan Intervention For Endpoint reduction in hypertension study (LIFE): A randomised trial against atenolol. *Lancet.* 2002;359:995–1003.

52. North American Symptomatic Carotid Endarterectomy Trial Collaborators. Beneficial effect of carotid endarterectomy in symptomatic patients with high-grade carotid stenosis. *N Engl J Med.* 1991;325:445–453.

53. Barnett HJ, Taylor DW, Eliasziw M, et al. Benefit of carotid endarterectomy in patients with symptomatic moderate or severe stenosis. North American Symptomatic Carotid Endarterectomy Trial Collaborators. *N Engl J Med.* 1998;339:1415–1425.

54. European Carotid Surgery Trialists' Collaborative Group. Randomised trial of endarterectomy for recently symptomatic carotid stenosis: final results of the MRC European Carotid Surgery Trial (ECST). *Lancet.* 1998;351:1379–1387.

55. Halliday A, Mansfield A, Marro J, et al. Prevention of disabling and fatal strokes by successful carotid

endarterectomy in patients without recent neurological symptoms: randomised controlled trial. *Lancet.* 2004; 363:1491–1502.

56. Wennberg DE, Lucas FL, Birkmeyer JD, Bredenberg CE, Fisher ES. Variation in carotid endarterectomy mortality in the Medicare population: Trial hospitals, volume, and patient characteristics. *JAMA.* 1998;279:1278–1281.

57. Sacco RL, Adams R, Albers G, et al. Guidelines for prevention of stroke in patients with ischemic stroke or transient ischemic attack: a statement for healthcare professionals from the American Heart Association/American Stroke Association Council on Stroke: Co-sponsored by the Council on Cardiovascular Radiology and Intervention: the American Academy of Neurology affirms the value of this guideline. *Stroke.* 2006;37:577–617.

58. McCabe DJ, Pereira AC, Clifton A, Bland JM, Brown MM, CAVATAS Investigators. Restenosis after carotid angioplasty, stenting, or endarterectomy in the Carotid and Vertebral Artery Transluminal Angioplasty Study (CAVATAS). *Stroke.* 2005;36:281–286.

59. Alberts MJ. Results of a multicenter prospective randomized trial of carotid artery stenting vs. carotid endarterectomy (abstr). *Stroke.* 2001;32:325.

60. Alberts MJ, McCann R, Smith TP, et al. A randomized trial of carotid stenting vs. endarterectomy in patients with symptomatic carotid stenosis: study design. *J Neurovasc Dis.* 1997;2:228–234.

61. CARESS Steering Committee. Carotid revascularization using endarterectomy or stenting systems (CARESS): phase I clinical trial. *J Endovasc Ther.* 2003;10:1021–1030.

62. CaRESS Steering Committee. Carotid Revascularization Using Endarterectomy or Stenting Systems (CaRESS) phase I clinical trial: 1-year results. *J Vasc Surg.* 2005;42: 213–219.

63. Yadav JS, Wholey MH, Kuntz RE, et al. Protected carotid-artery stenting versus endarterectomy in high-risk patients. *N Engl J Med.* 2004;351:1493–1501.

64. SPACE Collaborative Group, Ringleb PA, Allenberg J, et al. 30 day results from the SPACE trial of stent-protected angioplasty versus carotid endarterectomy in symptomatic patients: a randomised non-inferiority trial. *Lancet.* 2006;368:1239–1247.

65. Mas JL, Chatellier G, Beyssen B, et al. Endarterectomy versus stenting in patients with symptomatic severe carotid stenosis. *N Engl J Med.* 2006;355:1660–1671.

66. Kastrup A, Nagele T, Groschel K, et al. Incidence of new brain lesions after carotid stenting with and without cerebral protection. *Stroke.* 2006;37:2312–2316.

67. Lacroix V, Hammer F, Astarci P, et al. Ischemic cerebral lesions after carotid surgery and carotid stenting. *Eur J Vasc Endovasc Surg.* 2007;33:430–435.

68. Biller J, Feinberg WM, Castaldo JE, et al. Guidelines for carotid endarterectomy: a statement for healthcare professionals from a Special Writing Group of the Stroke Council, American Heart Association. *Circulation.* 1998;97:501–509.

69. Hobson RW, 2nd, Mackey WC, Ascher E, et al. Management of atherosclerotic carotid artery disease: clinical practice guidelines of the Society for Vascular Surgery. *J Vasc Surg.* 2008;48:480–486.

70. Levy EI, Mocco J, Samuelson RM, Ecker RD, Jahromi BS, Hopkins LN. Optimal treatment of carotid artery disease. *J Am Coll Cardiol.* 2008;51:979–985.

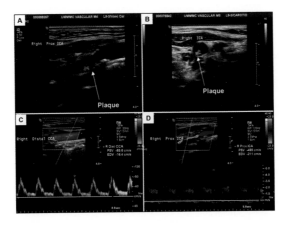

Plate 7

Figure 6.8 Carotid ultrasound in a patient with significant carotid artery stenosis. Panel A: Longitudinal two-dimensional view of the internal carotid artery reveals large heterogeneous plaque burden. Panel B: Transverse two-dimensional view of the same carotid with atherosclerotic plaque. Panel C: Color and spectral Doppler of the distal common carotid artery (proximal to the stenotic segment) reveal laminar blood flow and normal flow velocity. Panel D: Color Doppler of the proximal right internal carotid artery reveals color aliasing suggestive of turbulent flow; spectral Doppler shows an increased velocity of 4.8 meters per second, and a persistent diastolic flow gradient, consistent with severe carotid stenosis.

Images courtesy of Denise Kush, RDMS, RVT; Vascular Laboratory, UMass Memorial Health Care.

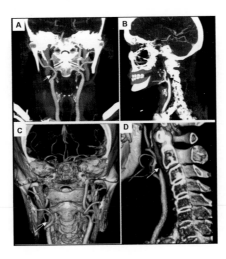

Plate 8

Figure 6.10 Computed tomography angiography in a patient with right internal carotid artery occlusion. Panel A: Coronal two-dimensional maximum intensity projection (MIP) view. Panel B: Sagittal two-dimensional MIP view. Panel C: Coronal three-dimensional reconstruction. Panel D: Sagittal three-dimensional reconstruction. Arrows indicate site of occlusion of the right internal carotid artery.

Figures courtesy of David J. Sheehan, DO; Radiology Department, University of Massachusetts Medical Center and Medical School.

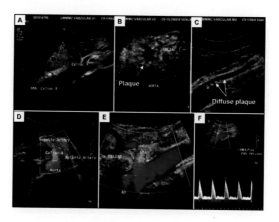

Plate 5

Figure 4.4 Duplex ultrasound of the celiac and mesenteric vessels. Panel A: Two-dimensional longitudinal view of the aorta at the origin of the celiac and superior mesenteric artery (SMA). Panel B: Transverse two-dimensional view of the aorta reveals calcified plaque at the origin of the celiac artery. Panel C: Longitudinal two-dimensional view of a superior mesenteric artery with diffuse calcified plaque. Panel D: Transverse two-dimensional and color Doppler view of the aorta at the level of the celiac artery and its bifurcation into the hepatic and splenic arteries. Panel E: Longitudinal two-dimensional and color Doppler view of the aorta at the level of the celiac and SMA origin. Panel F: Normal color and spectral Doppler profile in the superior mesenteric artery.

Images courtesy of Denise Kush, RDMS, RVT; Vascular Laboratory, UMass Memorial Health Care.

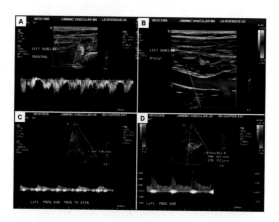

Plate 6

Figure 5.10 Subclavian arterial Duplex ultrasound. Panels A and B: Two-dimensional, spectral and color Doppler of a normal proximal and distal left subclavian artery. Panel C: Color and spectral Doppler of the left subclavian proximal to a stenotic segment reveal normal flow. Panel D: Color Doppler distal to a stenotic segment reveals aliasing, suggestive of turbulent flow; spectral Doppler indicates increased velocity of 4.2 meters per second, consistent with significant subclavian stenosis.

Images courtesy of Denise Kush, RDMS, RVT; Vascular Laboratory, UMass Memorial Health Care.

Plate   C-3

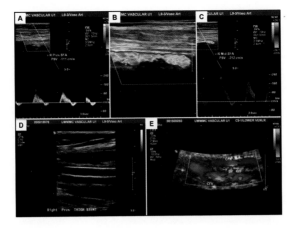

Plate 3

Figure 2.17 Duplex ultrasound of the lower extremities. Panels A to C: Normal velocity in the superficial femoral artery (Panel A) proximal to a stenosis that produces color aliasing due to turbulent flow (Panel B) and an intra- and post-stenotic increase in flow velocity distal to the stenosis (Panel C). Panel D: Two-dimensional ultrasound of a patent superficial femoral artery stent. Panel E: Iatrogenic arteriovenous fistula (AVF, arteriovenous fistula; CFA, common femoral artery; CFV, common femoral vein; arrow indicates the fistulous communication).

Images courtesy of Denise Kush, RDMS, RVT; Vascular Laboratory, UMass Memorial Health Care.

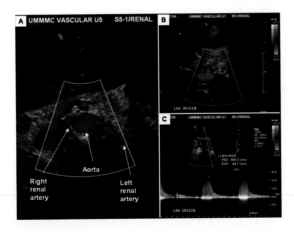

Plate 4

Figure 3.5 Renal duplex ultrasound. Panel A: Normal two-dimensional and color Doppler transverse view of the aorta at the origin of the renal arteries with non-turbulent flow. Panel B: Two-dimensional and color Doppler transverse view of the left renal artery in a patient with significant atherosclerotic renal artery stenosis; arrows indicate heavily calcified plaque in the proximal segment. Panel C: Color and spectral Doppler of the left renal artery show an increased velocity of 50 meters per second in the proximal left renal artery, consistent with severe renal artery stenosis.

Images courtesy of Denise Kush, RDMS, RVT; Vascular Laboratory, UMass Memorial Health Care.

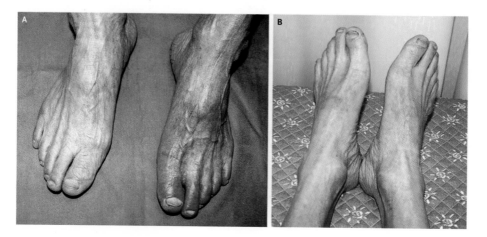

Plate 1

Figure 2.11 Photographs of common physical exam findings in a patient with claudication. In panel A, the left foot is erythematous, cold to touch, and pulseless in the dorsalis pedis and posterior tibial artery territories, while hanging down. In panel B, the foot becomes pale when the extremities are elevated. This is consistent with Buerger's sign, suggestive of peripheral artery disease.

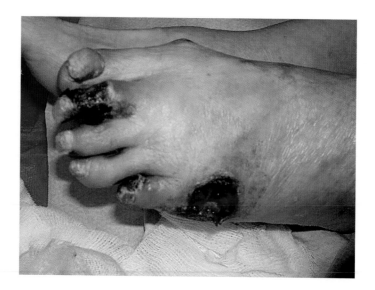

Plate 2

Figure 2.12 Critical limb ischemia. There is rubor of the forefoot, gangrene of the digits, and an ulceration.

Plate C-1